P9-CFT-917

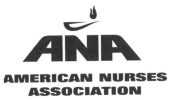

AMERICAN NURSES
ASSOCIATION

NURSING ADMINISTRATION:
SCOPE AND STANDARDS
OF PRACTICE

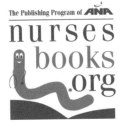

The Publishing Program of ANA

nurses
books
.org

AMERICAN NURSES ASSOCIATION
SILVER SPRING, MARYLAND
2009

Library of Congress Cataloging-in-Publication data

Nursing administration : scope and standards of practice / American Nurses Association.
   p. ; cm.
   Includes bibliographical references and index.
   ISBN-13: 978-1-55810-267-5 (pbk.)
   ISBN-10: 1-55810-267-1 (pbk.)
   1. Nurse administrators. 2. Nursing services—Administration. I. American Nurses Association.
   [DNLM: 1. Nurse Administrators—standards. 2. Nursing Care—standards.
3. Professional Competence—standards. WY 105 N97419 2009]

RT89.N73 2009
362.17'3068—dc22   2009008708

The American Nurses Association (ANA) is a national professional association. This ANA publication—*Nursing Administration: Scope and Standards of Practice*—reflects the thinking of the nursing profession on various issues and should be reviewed in conjunction with state board of nursing policies and practices. State law, rules, and regulations govern the practice of nursing, while *Nursing Administration: Scope and Standards of Practice* guides nurses in the application of their professional skills and responsibilities.

Published by Nursesbooks.org
The Publishing Program of ANA

American Nurses Association
8515 Georgia Avenue, Suite 400
Silver Spring, MD 20910-3492
1-800-274-4ANA
http://www.Nursesbooks.org/

The ANA is the only full-service professional organization representing the interests of the nation's 2.9 million registered nurses through its 53 constituent member nurses associations, its 24 specialty nursing and workforce advocacy affiliate organizations that currently connect to ANA as affiliates. The ANA advances the nursing profession by fostering high standards of nursing practice, promoting the rights of nurses in the workplace, projecting a positive and realistic view of nursing, and by lobbying the Congress and regulatory agencies on healthcare issues affecting nurses and the public.

Design: Scott Bell, Arlington, VA ~ Freedom by Design, Alexandria, VA ~ Stacy Maguire, Sterling, VA ~ *Project Management & Editing*: Eric Wurzbacher, ANA staff ~ *Copyediting*: Lisa Anthony, Chapel Hill, NC ~ *Proofreading*: Ashley Mason, Atlanta GA ~ *Indexing*: Estalita Slivoskey, Havre de Grace, MD ~ *Composition*: House of Equations, Inc., Arden, NC *Printing*: McArdle Printing, Upper Marlboro, MD

© 2009 American Nurses Association. All rights reserved. No part of this book may be reproduced or utilized in any form or any means, electronic or mechanical, including photocopying and recording, or by any information storage and retrieval system, without permission in writing from the publisher.

First printing April 2009.

ISBN-13: 978-1-55810-267-5   SAN: 851-3481   10M   04/09

Acknowledgments

Work Group Members

Lynne Bill, MS, RN, CNAA-BC

Judy Lentz, MSN, RN, NHA

Joy F. Reed, EdD, RN, FAAN

Kenneth Rempher, PhD, MBA, RN, CCRN, APRN-BC

Pauline F. Robitaille, MSN, RN, CNOR

Chris Weigel, MBA, BSN, RN

American Nurses Association Staff

Carol J. Bickford, PhD, RN-BC – Content editor

Katherine C. Brewer, MSN, RN – Content editor

Yvonne Humes, MSA – Project coordinator

Maureen E. Cones, Esq. – Legal counsel

CONTENTS

SCOPE AND STANDARDS OF NURSING ADMINISTRATION PRACTICE

Function of the Scope of Practice Statement

The scope of practice statement (pages 1–23) describes the "who","what", "where","when","why" and "how" of nursing practice. Each of these questions must be sufficiently answered to provide a complete picture of the practice and its boundaries and membership. The depth and breadth in which individual registered nurses engage in the total scope of nursing practice is dependent upon education, experience, role, and the population served.

Function of Standards

The standards, which are comprised of the standards of practice (pages 25–33) and the standards of professional performance (pages 35–44), are authoritative statements by which nurses practicing within the role, population, and specialty governed by this document (*Nursing Administration: Scope and Standards of Practice*) and describe the duties that they are expected to competently perform. The standards published herein may be utilized as evidence of the legal standard of care governing nurses practicing within the role, population, and specialty governed by this document. The standards are subject to change with the dynamics of the nursing profession and as new patterns of professional practice are developed and accepted by the nursing profession and the public. In addition, specific conditions and clinical circumstances may also affect the application of the standards at a given time; such as during a natural disaster. The standards are subject to formal, periodic review and revision.

The measurement criteria that appear below each standard are not all-inclusive and do not establish the legal standard of care. Rather, the measurement criteria are specific, measurable elements that can be used by nursing professionals to measure professional performance. Nurses practicing within this particular role, population, and specialty can identify opportunities for development and improvement by evaluating performance on these elements.

PREFACE

Nursing Administration: Scope and Standards of Practice reflects the significant evolution of the standards of practice for the nurse administrator in comparison to those standards first presented in the original American Nurses Association (ANA) 1991 publication, *Standards for Organized Nursing Services and Responsibilities of Nurse Administrators Across All Settings*, and those included in later editions. Similarly, this nursing administration scope of practice statement differs greatly from both the original language in the 1995 *Scope and Standards for Nurse Administrators* and as revised in its 2004 edition. The expanded content and new format are intended to best describe who the nurse administrators are, where they practice, and how they influence the healthcare environment and organization. This scope of practice statement moves away from the traditional view of nurse administrators as either the nurse executive or the nurse manager and attempts to reflect the diversity of this specialty nursing practice, emphasizing the variety and dimensions of leadership and oversight that characterize nursing administration. As a professional resource, this new edition also contains a more robust examination of literature and identifies practice frameworks that are becoming more prevalent as nurse administrators address contemporary and future issues and trends. This is a departure from the previous versions, which were more focused on the levels and qualifications of nurse administrators.

This document is the product of the discussions and thinking of a small work group of nurse administrators from diverse specialty and practice settings. Their original draft document submitted for an extended public comment period generated recommendations for revisions. The work group then completed its final draft and submitted that work to the two-tiered ANA review process: examination first by the Committee on Nursing Practice Standards and Guidelines of the Congress on Nursing Practice and Economics (CNPE) and then by the CNPE as a whole. The additional revisions recommended by these bodies were integrated into the final draft for publication.

Additional Content

For a better appreciation of the historical and professional context underlying *Nursing Administration: Scope and Standards of Practice*, the content of *Scope and Standards for Nurse Administrators* (2004) has been reproduced in Appendix B (starting on page 49) and is indexed with the current content of this edition. That 2004 work was the immediate predecessor to this current edition.

NURSING ADMINISTRATION SCOPE OF PRACTICE

Function of the Scope of Practice Statement

The scope of practice statement (pages 1–23) describes the "who", "what", "where", "when", "why" and "how" of nursing practice. Each of these questions must be sufficiently answered to provide a complete picture of the practice and its boundaries and membership. The depth and breadth in which individual registered nurses engage in the total scope of nursing practice is dependent upon education, experience, role, and the population served.

Introduction

Nursing is a dynamic profession, with nurses engaged in various health-care roles related to planning, education, research, systems, and the promotion, maintenance, and improvement of health. Nurses find themselves in a private or public healthcare industry that calls on creativity, innovation, flexibility, and endurance to overcome barriers and create a healthy work environment. Thus, nursing administration as a specialty mirrors that diversity, as almost every nursing service requires some kind of leadership and oversight. This role specialty encompasses the full spectrum of nursing practice and settings.

Nurse administrators emerge as representatives of their profession and advocates for nursing and healthcare systems that provide excellence in care and improve health, patient safety, and quality. These administrators utilize creative and intelligent leadership skills and strategies to guide registered nurses in their professional work, establish and maintain supportive and enabling environments for nursing practice, and support their organization or institution. Nurse administrators within private healthcare and public sectors can foster a collaborative approach to nursing education, mentoring and inspiring those who work around them, appreciating the need for attention to organizational systems, and instilling a sense of interdisciplinary participation in all levels of care.

Health care proves to be a complex industry, with ever-changing public expectations, new regulations, scarce resources and increased service demands, and environmental concerns. As the American population ages and an entire generation enters Medicare eligibility, health care will continue along this trend, and demand for healthcare services will be greater than ever. That, coupled with a continuing nursing shortage and aging workforce, has been described as the perfect storm (Curtin, 2007). Well-prepared nurse administrators provide the requisite leadership to lead nurses and other interprofessional healthcare personnel through the storm, and enhance health care and the health of populations into the coming decades.

Nurse administrators project a shared vision for the future of nursing and of the healthcare industry. They face the challenges of complicated healthcare delivery systems by demonstrating effective leadership, developing creative strategic plans for nursing practice and care, and providing solutions to healthcare problems by enhancing and elevating the work of the nursing profession.

Effective and dynamic leadership by nurse administrators will help develop well-planned organizational structures, inclusive decision-making, creative and supportive personnel policies, and professional models of care that promote excellent services. Such leadership promotes collegial interdisciplinary relationships and the professional growth and development of nursing staff. The impact and effectiveness of such leadership will influence public policy and determine the future role of nursing in an evolving healthcare environment.

Definition of Nurse Administrators

Broadly defined, the nurse administrator is a registered nurse who orchestrates and influences the work of others in a defined environment, most often healthcare focused, to enhance the shared vision of an organization or institution. Due to the dynamism of the healthcare industry, nurse administrators direct a wide array of nursing practice in clinical and non-clinical settings. While nurse administrators are present in many forms and at various levels, certain global themes permeate all roles, including advocacy, leadership, shared vision, knowledge of business practices and processes, mentorship, and dedication to the profession. The goals of the nurse administrator's efforts are a quality product focused on safety and the requisite infrastructures that seek to meet the expectations of the nursing profession, the consumer, and society.

The role of the nurse administrator is multifaceted and requires broad-level thinking. The nurse administrator is nimble in understanding and balancing business duties and obligations with the ongoing commitment to nursing. This dichotomy can cause tensions or even conflicts of interest, as nurse administrators seek to enhance quality nursing practice in organizations with values that may not always reflect those of nursing. However, even as corporate employees, administrators must act as registered nurses first by upholding the values of nursing and advocating for those values to the utmost extent possible.

Although nurse administrators are the most visible leaders in their defined roles, all nurses need to understand and embrace the competencies of nursing leadership. Nurses should also know what competencies to expect from their nurse administrators. Every nurse is a leader in some way, whether to colleagues, patients, students, or the community. Therefore every nurse should be aware of and exemplify leadership skills and traits.

Importance and Value of Nurse Administrators

Nurse administrators have the responsibility to address nursing practice both internally and externally. This means they deal with issues on the employee or student level and address issues that affect delivery of services to their consumers. They foster openness, interdisciplinary collaboration, and accountability in colleagues and those they direct or supervise. They create an environment that facilitates and encourages nursing staff to demonstrate accountability for their own practice. Such an environment empowers registered nurses at all levels of the organization to synthesize knowledge, use critical thinking, and participate in decision-making that affects their practice. Nurse administrators help define the values of the organization, facility, or team; foster collaboration, communication, and goal-setting; and strive for excellence among and across the continuum of care and the populations they work with or affect.

Nurse administrators establish the environment that gives nurses a voice in the decision-making process and permits organizational, departmental, and unit-based decisions to meet the needs and expectations of all stakeholders affected by those decisions. They advocate for the needs of nurses and seek resources, including funding, technologies, and staff, to meet those needs. They champion outcome measures and metrics that place value on nursing, both in terms of quality and cost-effectiveness.

Nurse administrators actively partner with others to incorporate new technologies that enhance nursing work, recruit experts to provide staff support, and devise ways to change and improve processes. This advocacy role is uniquely implemented by nurse administrators through use of their authority and power to maintain the integrity of their own nursing practice and the practice of other nurses or staff under their purview. Nurse administrators demonstrate trust in the ability of nurses to work independently to achieve a common goal. This allows nurses and other employees to work according to their personal and professional preferences while maintaining adherence to pertinent considerations (e.g., professional ethics, regulations).

Nurse administrators shape the environment in which nurses practice and teach and consumers receive health care, with the goal of inspiring those around them to reach for excellence in their practice. Nurse administrators act as mentors to those around them, helping assure that nurses develop from novice to expert in a safe, comfortable, supportive environment, and at their own pace without feeling rushed or fearing making mistakes. Nurse administrators must create an environment where nurses feel comfortable informing leadership of situations or incidents that compromise or threaten quality care delivery, and where mistakes or other incidences are viewed as opportunities to improve systems, not as occurrences mandating punishment or blame of individuals. Nurse administrators themselves seek opportunities to continue their journey to become expert in their roles, and they can identify and remedy their own shortcomings.

Employee satisfaction, successful recruitment and retention efforts, quality outcomes, and elevation of the image of nursing practice are metrics often used to determine the success of the nurse administrator. The nurse administrator also seeks direct feedback from staff on his or her performance. Their personal diligence and drive to achieve excellence and quality in their practice inspire the work of nurses or other personnel they direct, thus contributing to the overall success of the practice or business they direct. The success and commitment to excellence of nurses in an organization speaks highly of the leadership example set by the nurse administrator.

Frameworks for Practice

Nurse administrators at all levels and in all types of settings share common frameworks that guide practice in achieving goals. These frameworks should support the nurse administrator's diverse skills in organizational analysis, strategic planning, quality enhancement, and patient safety. How nurse administrator positions are made operational also depends upon the surrounding context, including organizational structure and complexity of the settings. The following frameworks are exemplars and do not constitute an exhaustive list.

Nursing Process

Nurse administrators draw on their nursing and business skills as they perform in their roles. They achieve outcomes by building on the nursing process, with its assessment, diagnosis, outcomes identification, planning, implementation, and evaluation components, and melding that into a traditional business process. This creates a hybrid system of management and function, but one that nurses recognize and understand. Nurse administrators make decisions based on evidence and data wherever possible, and also rely on experience and intuition to inform their decisions.

Culture of Quality and Safety

The nurse administrator strives to create an environment where nursing and other services are delivered safely and effectively. The creation of such an environment arises from the ethical and social obligations of nurses to deliver safe, quality services, and also from the need to simultaneously protect the organization and its employees from failure and liability. Nurse administrators, as representatives of nursing and also stewards to the organization, must leverage their decision-making to employ critical thinking, problem-solving techniques, and collaboration skills to design systems that promote quality outcomes, minimize risk, and appeal to all organization stakeholders—nurses, organizational leadership, healthcare and other professionals, investors and funding sources, and the healthcare consumer.

However, creating a system of quality and safety requires creating an entire culture of safety. Nurse administrators should promote a process of mistake or error mitigation that recognizes that errors may be the result of system breakdowns or failures to build a good system, as opposed to putting the total blame on individuals. Such a culture focuses on investigation of the root cause of an incident, addresses necessary system(s) modification, and reserves punitive action for reckless behavior. The system promotes reporting and quality outcomes, which ultimately can reduce cost, promote transparency and public trust, and make nurses accountable for their practice. Three reports from the Institute of Medicine provide insight and rationale for improving safety and quality: *To Err Is Human: Building A Safer Health System* (1999), *Patient Safety: Achieving A New Standard of Care* (2003a), and *Keeping Patients Safe: Transforming the Work Environment of Nurses* (2003b). These reports brought significant attention to the idea of treating errors as systems failures. One model for error prevention and mitigation is the Just Culture approach, a process garnering increased interest in healthcare settings because of its focus on fixing error-prone systems by supporting error reporting, error reduction, and patient safety (Asiton & Chou, 2005).

Appreciative Inquiry

Appreciative inquiry is both a philosophy and methodology that promotes the positive aspects of past or present work environments, can be used to promote change management, and can be incorporated into communication or process improvement initiatives (Havens, Wood, & Leeman, 2006). Appreciative inquiry builds on the premise that positive work environments result from focus on the successes and positive aspects of current processes, systems, or work culture, accompanied with maximum replication and enhancement. Administrators can use appreciative inquiry in complex, organization-wide projects or simply promote its use among individual units of staff.

Organizational Development Resources

Nurse administrators function as an organizational development resource, whether part of a small staff, a large company, a product development initiative, or one's own entrepreneurial enterprise. This requires understanding of human resources theories and how to best tap the talents and abilities of the people that make up the organization's workforce. The administrator uses this lens to mitigate problems in the work environment, encourage problem solving, meet the needs of employees, and enable and inspire employees to achieve their full potential.

Mentoring

Nurse administrators also function as mentors. This reflects the current trend in workforce development and management of approaching employees as coaches first, and bosses second. The nurse administrator who directs staff must understand their needs and how they best respond to management. Nurse administrators lead without fear and inspire their staff to appreciate and accept change. They encourage and engage them to be part of that change process. Embracing cultural diversity and acceptance of nurses' rights to govern themselves are paramount to achieving a successful work environment for nurses.

Emotional Intelligence

Emotional intelligence is an important skill set and attitude measurement for administrators. This involves demonstrated commitment to teambuilding, communication, relationship management, fostering change, understanding and respecting workplace culture, inspiration for colleagues, and balance of emotions and interests (Carroll, 2005). Nurse administrators encourage feedback from others when assessing their own performance and attitudes, and seek opportunities to improve. They demonstrate self-management in controlling negative emotions, display honesty and integrity, model flexibility and adaptability in changing situations, and exhibit a keen sense of reality. Nurse administrators proactively respond to trends and situations in their organizations or consumer base and capitalize on opportunities to promote beneficial change, outcome improvement, or other enhancements of the work environment or workforce.

Transformational Leadership

As originally described by Burns (1978), transformational leadership provides a framework for leaders and managers in dealing with those who work for them. Transformational leaders foster open communication horizontally and vertically, provide inspiration and enthusiasm, and create harmony among staff. They seek to improve communication, staff satisfaction, and output (Robbins & Davidhizar, 2007). Within this framework, nurse administrators define and project shared vision, demonstrate dedication and continued commitment on the journey toward a vision, motivate and contribute to positive change, give individualized attention to staff, and allow for shared decision-making (Rearick, 2007). This leadership guides those working in such an environment to find greater meaning in their tasks, and as a result share responsibility and dedication to quality. Transformational leadership sharply contrasts with a more transactional, operational view of work.

Servant Leadership

Servant leadership is a theory of leadership in which the leader acts entirely on the behalf of those led (Greenleaf, 1978). Using 10 key principles, the leader engages and enhances those they lead to ultimately produce a quality outcome and an energized work environment. Servant leadership exploits the talents and abilities of individual members of a group, instead of dominating or controlling actions as in traditional models of hierarchical leadership (Neill & Saunders, 2008). For nurse administrators, servant leadership puts focus on the natural instincts of nurses to care for, respect, and value those under their purview, which enhances the nurses' confidence in providing care.

Magnet Recognition Program: 5 Model Components

Nurse administrators embrace the concepts reflected in the *Five Model Components* associated with the Magnet Recognition Program®: Transformational Leadership; Structural Empowerment; Exemplary Professional Practice; New Knowledge, Innovation, and Improvements; and Empirical Quality Results. They seek to provide the nurses and others in their facilities, organizations, schools, or agencies with the tools and skills necessary to achieve quality work (American Nurses Credentialing Center, 2008). This puts focus on recruiting and retaining quality staff, providing quality care or healthcare products, and valuing and enhancing the nursing profession. The *Five Model Components* can guide and direct quality work and enhance the profession wherever nurses practice.

Practice Environments

Nurse administrators can be found anywhere nurses work or where a healthcare product is created to serve the public or a specific consumer. They are instrumental in engaging staff to use critical thinking skills and strive for excellence in their work. Nurse administrators make decisions that guide nursing practice, set strategic goals, improve the work environment, and create and influence institutional and public policy. They advocate for their staff in the procurement and use of new technologies, evidence-based practice, human resources, policy decisions, funding, budgeting, environmental health principles, population-based approaches, or any factor that affects those that work with them or for them. Their nimble capacity allows them to be active parts of both the nursing and business sides of the practice environments. Such flexibility and dedication enhance the work environment around them.

Nursing administration practice occurs in a wide variety of settings, from private enterprises to the public sector, in large or small healthcare facilities, integrated delivery systems, corporate healthcare companies, professional organizations, academic settings, research facilities, government agencies, communities, correctional institutions, military healthcare entities, and other facilities.

While traditional roles in all healthcare settings continue to offer career growth, the areas where nurse administrators practice is ever expanding. New opportunities have been created with the expansion of responsibilities for multiple patient care services. At the corporate systems level in integrated care organizations, nurse administrators are structuring and planning nursing care systems across a complex continuum of services in multiple settings. In the public arena, nurses are increasingly collaborating with community partners to expand population-focused services, requiring nurse administrators to orchestrate and foster such collaborations. In academic settings, nurse administrators develop innovations in research, practice, and education; advocate for increased visibility; and enhance the image and importance of nursing within the institution and to the community at large. Nurses are often in the forefront leading government and organizational disaster planning and emergency response initiatives. These roles offer new challenges for nurse administrators and demand flexibility and creative vision.

Ethics

Nurse administrators in private and public settings are increasingly confronted with balancing the goals of nursing, goals of the organization, health of the population, and the health of the planet. Nurse administrators are constantly challenged to devise creative solutions to the dilemma of having to do more with fewer staff and other resources, without violating nursing or other professional ethics, environmental principles, institutional policy, or healthcare regulations.

Nurse administrators have a duty to advocate for nursing ethics as set out in ANA's *Code of Ethics for Nurses with Interpretive Statements* (2001). Even in the smallest arenas, nurse administrators are vital resources in maintaining, respecting, and upholding the provisions of the code of ethics for nursing, as well as the nursing and specialty nursing scope of practice statements and standards of practice. Such actions both protect and enhance the nursing work that they oversee or complete themselves, guaranteeing a safe, quality, effective product for the consumers of that work effort.

Legal and Regulatory Compliance

Nurse administrators must understand and abide by federal, state, and local laws and regulations pertaining to the practices under their auspice. Upholding nurse practice acts, verifying and tracking licensure and credentialing of all applicable staff, abiding by nurses' rights, and compliance with regulatory and professional standards are duties of the nurse administrator at any level. Federal and state law may also dictate quality and practice standards. Nurse administrators should use applicable legal standards as opportunities to promote safe, quality, nurse-centered delivery systems.

Key Elements of the Nurse Administrator Role

Of key importance, nurse administrators strive to represent the quality work from nurses or other healthcare personnel under their direction.

At any level, nurse administrators promote:

- Accountability for nursing practice
- Clinical and workplace autonomy for nurses
- Nursing control of nursing practice and oversight of the practice environment
- Respect for nurses' rights and responsibilities
- Open communication between staff and administration
- Positive working relationships among the healthcare team
- A safe and healthy workplace
- Evidence-based practice
- Adequate compensation commensurate with responsibilities, education, and experience
- Adequate numbers of clinically competent staff
- Access to education, research, and appropriate technologies
- Care that satisfies the healthcare consumer
- Stewardship of allocated resources.

Spheres of Influence

In past versions of the nursing administration scope and standards of practice, nurse administrators were identified and titled as Nurse Executive and Nurse Manager. This revision provides a different approach and seeks to classify nurse administrators by their level of oversight or sphere of influence. This approach seems to provide a more accurate classification of administrators than job titles. However, the nurse administrator operates in a work continuum, and it is difficult to fit every administrator into only one category. Their individual key elements or job requirements might put them in more than one sphere of influence; they might fall between spheres in a middle management role, or they might find the sphere of influence is applicable even though they are not in a role defined as administration. These spheres include, but are not limited to: organization-wide, unit-based or service-line-based, program-focused, and project- or specific task-based authority.

Organization-wide Authority

Nurse administrators with organization-wide authority represent the ultimate nursing authority at the top organizational leadership level. They are tasked with the overall management of all nursing practice and services and most often assume organizational titles such as Chief Nursing Officer (CNO), Director of Nursing Services, Dean, or Bureau Chief. Increasing numbers of nurse administrators at this level are moving into other senior leadership or executive positions, such as Chief Executive Officer or Chief Operating Officer.

The main element of their practice is to understand and respond to the needs of the organization, as well as maintain the organization's communication with a greater oversight body. In private institutions, this body might be the board of trustees, board of directors, investors, or stockholders. However in the public sector, the oversight body might be department or agency leadership, a legislative body, or taxpayers. These nurse administrators hold the authority to manage within the context of the organization as a whole and to transform organizational values into daily operations yielding an efficient, effective, environmentally healthy, and caring organization. This authority is exercised globally across the organization's delivery systems and across the care continuum.

At this level, a nurse administrator serves as a catalyst and role model, providing leadership and direction in accord with both the organization's mission and values and nursing's core ideology. Collaboration and partnering are necessary to share and nourish this ideology, to foster better relationships across organizations, practices, interest groups, and the community, and thus achieve better communication and outcomes.

The nurse administrator at this level demonstrates attention to strategic planning, provides a strong voice for nursing at the overall institutional management level, and gains respect for nursing practice. He or she promotes the evidence-based model in policy and program development, implementation, and evaluation, and monitors policies and decisions regarding nursing practice for adherence to applicable professional standards and practice guidelines. The nurse administrator at this level provides a professional nursing practice environment in which registered nurses have control over nursing practice and autonomy in their workplace (Weston, 2008). Nurses engaged in shared governance are empowered to provide effective, efficient, safe, and compassionate quality care and have opportunities for ongoing professional growth and development.

Drawing on a model developed by the American Organization of Nurse Executives (AONE, 2005), nurse administrators at organizational helms should blend business competencies and skills with the core ideology of nursing. This allows the nurse administrator to integrate the nursing process into business decisions. He or she also collaborates in the organization-wide healthcare delivery system and process design. These efforts include advocacy for a safe and healthy physical work environment through the implementation of such things as nursing workload measurement, clinical and financial projection models based on healthcare economics, data collection and analysis, outcomes identification and measurement, practice innovations, and recruitment and retention initiatives. Nurse administrators at this level have a key role in assigning value to and advocating for implementation and funding of greater use of technologies to improve physical work elements, protect nurses, enhance quality, and streamline processes.

In any organization, these nurse administrators provide leadership in professional, community, and legislative initiatives to help shape the future of nursing, healthcare policy, and societal health overall. They advocate for transparency of nursing administration, respect for nurses' rights and responsibilities, and provide a work environment for nurses free from physical, psychological, or emotional abuse. They promote adequate communication between staff and management and be-tween the organization and the public, and they lead the organization to strive for quality service.

Characteristics of the role of the nurse with organization-wide authority include, but are not limited to:

- Supporting the notion that professional nurses should govern their practice;

- Participating in the leadership of the healthcare organization as a full member of the executive team;

- Providing leadership in the strategic planning of the healthcare or-ganization and nursing;

- Actively guiding the nursing profession to its objectives, such as those in *Nursing's Agenda for the Future* (ANA, 2001);

- Providing leadership in the determination of clinical, scholarly, and administrative nursing goals and directions, as well as the associ-ated functions and processes necessary to achieve those goals;

- Acquiring and allocating human, material, and financial resources for specific functions and processes;

- Evaluating and revising systems and processes of nursing services that achieve nurse-sensitive patient-, client-, or family-centered outcomes;

- Providing leadership in knowledge synthesis, critical thinking, problem solving, managing conflict, and addressing ethical issues;

- Providing leadership in human resource development and management;

- Providing opportunities for consumer input into personal health-care decisions and policy development;

- Establishing ongoing evaluation and innovation of services pro-vided by nursing services and the organization as a whole;

- Facilitating the conduct, dissemination, and utilization of research to create evidence-based nursing, health care, management and administrative systems;

- Serving as a professional role model and mentor to motivate, develop, recruit, and retain future nurse administrators;

- Serving as an agent of change, assisting all staff in understanding the importance, necessity, impact, and process of change;
- Constructing a nursing workforce that reflects population diversity;
- Promoting the delivery of culturally competent care;
- Supporting outcome measurement and evidence-based practice;
- Allocating resources based on patient need for nursing care;
- Encouraging registered nurse participation in decision-making at varied levels of the organization;
- Integrating appropriate technologies to meet the needs of professional nursing and enhance patient and nurse safety;
- Providing a work environment that is physically, emotionally, and psychologically safe for nurses and others to practice;
- Increasing the educational preparation of the nurse workforce;
- Actively participating in the institution's emergency planning;
- Communicating effectively with staff;
- Responding to expressed needs from staff and providing leadership by example; and
- Maintaining professional development programs that support and enhance the development and maintenance of professional competence and the requisite associated competencies.

Unit-Based or Service-Line-based Authority

Nurse administrators managing units of people are charged with handling the daily operations of a unit or service line and complete the face-to-face interaction and necessary work with staff. These nurse administrators may be assigned titles such as nurse manager, clinical coordinator, nursing supervisor, or patient care director. They may or may not be accountable to a nurse administrator at the organizational level.

At this level, nurse administrators advocate for and allocate available resources to promote efficient, effective, safe, and compassionate nursing care based on current standards of practice. They serve as the conduits between nurses and executive management, representing and advocating for their staff. Other responsibilities vary depending on the size and function of the organization.

These administrators coordinate activities between defined areas, providing clinical and administrative leadership and expertise. They facilitate an atmosphere of interactive management and the development of collegial relationships among nursing personnel and others. They serve as a link between nursing personnel and other healthcare disciplines and workers throughout the organization and within the healthcare community. These administrators have major roles in the implementation of the vision, mission, philosophy, core values, evidence-based practice, and standards of the organization.

These administrators are most visible in the environment in which nursing is practiced. They create a learning environment that is open, respectful, and promotes the sharing of expertise to promote the benefits of health outcomes. The ability of nurse managers to enhance the practice environment and professional development of nurses is critical to the recruitment and retention of registered nurses with diverse backgrounds and appropriate education and experience. They contribute to the strategic planning process, day-to-day operations, standards of care, and attainment of organizational goals . They collaborate with executive nurses and others in organizational planning, innovation, and evaluation. In larger organizations, the nurse manager may include further delineated levels.

Since their main work element is working with nurses directly, these administrators are responsible for their staff's actions and should also monitor and promote educational preparation of their staff on their individual roles in the healthcare setting. Oversight and management skills are crucial to provide effective leadership to staff to achieve desired patient or unit goals. These administrators must also understand and respect the specialty nursing scope and standards of practice of the nurses they manage, the state and federal laws regarding care provided in their units, and the policies of the facility or organization. These administrators should also establish appropriate orientation programs for all assigned staff.

Role characteristics of the nurse with unit-based or service-line-based authority include, but are not limited to:

- Promoting care delivery with respect for individuals' rights and preferences;
- Participating in nursing and organizational policy formulation and decision-making involving staff, such as in shared governance;
- Accepting organizational accountability for services provided to recipients;

- Evaluating the quality and appropriateness of health care;
- Coordinating nursing care with other healthcare disciplines, and assisting in integrating services across the continuum of health care;
- Participating in the recruitment, selection, and retention of personnel, including staff representative of the population diversity;
- Assessing impact of plans and strategies to address such issues as:
  - ethnic, cultural, and diversity changes in the population
  - political and social influences
  - financial and economic issues
  - the aging of society and demographic trends
  - ethical issues related to health care
  - environmental influences on health
- Assuming oversight for staffing, and scheduling personnel considering scope of practice, competencies, patient needs, and complexity of care;
- Providing appropriate orientation for new staff, and providing individual feedback on staff development and progress;
- Encouraging staff members to attain education, credentialing, and continuing professional development;
- Providing guidance for and supervision of personnel accountable to the nurse manager;
- Evaluating performance of personnel in a fair and transparent manner;
- Developing, implementing, and monitoring the budget for their defined area(s) of responsibility;
- Participating in and involving the nursing staff in evaluative research activities to promote evidence-based practice;
- Facilitating educational experiences for nursing and other students;
- Encouraging shared accountability for professional practice;
- Advocating for a work environment that minimizes work-related illness and injury;

- Reporting any injuries or safety hazards, and taking corrective action as quickly as possible;

- Providing an open forum of communication with staff, allowing them ample opportunities to discuss issues and seek guidance; and

- Understanding and complying with state and federal laws concerning the healthcare services and practice they manage, and complying with all facility regulations and policies.

Program-focused Authority

Nurse administrators might find themselves directing particular programs, projects, or work units that are not comprised of nurses, where they bring the nursing perspective, systems-thinking, and advocacy skills to whatever the work entails. These might be government programs; technology, research, or legal initiatives; or collaborative efforts with other health or non-health professionals. In this capacity, nurse administrators focus on completion of the project plan, achievement of quality outcomes, accountability to funding source or the consumer, maintenance of communication between the program's elements (workforce, funding source, consumer), and ethical delivery of services.

These nurses utilize the nursing process as a framework that contributes to completion of the program's work and provides a quality product. They bring a unique perspective and the fundamental elements of nursing leadership to a diverse work group, applying those skills and abilities to blend a multitude of views and move the stakeholders toward a common goal. These nurse administrators could also be directing nurses working in conjunction with a program or research center to guide policy, provide guidance to others in the profession or specialty, or influence legislative decisions.

Project- or Specific Task-based Authority

Nurse administrators with project or specific task-based authority focus mostly on an expressed support function or need as set forth by the organization or institution. These are clinical improvement roles that do not necessarily have direct patient care responsibilities. This could include elements of human resources, admissions processes, grant allocations, or communications and media. These nurse administrators focus their efforts on creating an evidence-based, ethical, sound approach to solve an expressed need from nursing or other areas of the organization. Such a focus could be nursing recruitment and retention, piloting a Magnet® application, orienting and educating staff, directing student admissions, fundraising, or developing and promoting professional and collegial relationships. The administrators in these areas apply nursing values and processes to complete a specific task or address an identified need.

While specific role characteristics have not been outlined for the program-based or project- or specific task-based authority descriptions, nurse administrators in these categories demonstrate a hybrid set of behaviors derived from those described as applicable to organization-wide and unit-based or service-line-based authorities.

Qualifications of Nurse Administrators

Given the expectations of leadership and accountability of the nurse administrator, it is important to define the licensure, education, and experience required. Nurse administrators at all levels and within all settings must hold an active registered nurse license and meet the requirements in the state in which they practice.

Education and Certification

A nurse administrator should have a graduate-level degree in a relevant field of management, nursing, policy, or administration. A doctoral degree in a relevant field is strongly recommended for those in organization-wide authority or executive levels of practice.

Nurse administrators are expected to seek professional certification in nursing administration or other relevant management or applicable specialties. Nurse administrators are role models for their staff in demonstrating continuing professional development and lifelong learning.

Knowledge, Skills, and Abilities

The experience backgrounds of professional nurses who serve as nurse administrators must include clinical and administrative practice, which enables these registered nurses to consistently fulfill the responsibilities inherent in their respective administrative roles. The list on the following page is representative, not exhaustive.

Representative knowledge, skills, and abilities of nurse administrators

Knowledge of:

Care management systems
Change management
Clinical practice guidelines, standards of care, and best practices
Consumer healthcare issues
Cultural diversity
Data management
Emergency planning and response
Environmental health principles
Fiscal management and financial outcomes
Health and public policy
Healthcare economics
Healthcare evaluation and outcome measures
Information technology trends
Law, regulation, and ethics
Management systems, processes, and analyses
Management theory
Marketing initiatives
Nursing research and other scholarly activities
Organizational behavior and development
Patient and employee safety regulations
Performance improvement
Practice innovation
Professional nursing practice
Professional practice environment
Standards of clinical nursing practice
Systems for patient safety
Trends in business practices

Skills in:

Budgeting and monetary management
Coaching and mentorship
Conflict negotiation and resolution
Conversation facilitation, including difficult conversations
Correcting poor performance
Customer service
Empowerment
Engaging and translating realities
Evaluating care and employee performance
Evidence-based and shared decision-making
Goal setting
Interpersonal, interdisciplinary, inter- and intra-organizational communication
Measurement of patient needs, outcomes, nursing workload
Mitigating anxiety and hostile situations
Networking
Recognition and improvement of personal failings
Self-management, observation, and analysis
Social competence
Strategic visioning and planning
Teambuilding
Technical competence

Abilities to:

Adapt with flexibility to situations, personalities, and tasks
Appreciate balance between personal and professional life
Be forward-looking and forward-thinking
Be self-observant
Commit to excellence
Dedicate oneself to learning for self and others
Demonstrate passion and commitment to professional life
Exhibit trustworthiness, honesty, integrity
Exhibit tolerance for cultural diversity and individual work style
Inspire and motivate others
Integrate ethical principles within practice

Issues and Trends

Similar to years past, the healthcare environment demands excellent services and care, despite limited resources and numbers of nursing staff. Healthcare facilities continue to see the consumer as the key to revenue and respectability, with a bulk of consumer satisfaction arising from nursing care. Information technology, direct-to-consumer advertising, complicated third-party payer systems, demand for accountability for health outcomes, and spiraling healthcare costs add to the complexity of the healthcare environment. Nurses must strive to attain a balance between providing quality outcomes and cost-effective care. Meanwhile, controlling healthcare costs remains a significant priority for institutions and organizations, giving nurses the opportunity to promote systemic improvements that reduce costs but don't negatively affect care.

The nursing workforce shortage has not abated, and nurse administrators find themselves with an ever-growing demand for nursing services, with limited staff to fill that need. Advertising and public awareness campaigns for the nursing profession have resulted in higher enrollment in nursing programs, causing an influx of new nurses into the healthcare field. Nurse administrators must be prepared to both recruit new workforce members and prevent rapid and frequent turnover of nursing staff. This mandates a dedication to proper orientation and workplace satisfaction for new staff in order to retain them, along with adherence to self-care initiatives and protection against working while fatigued.

One solution to the workforce shortage includes recruitment of internationally trained nurses. This presents nurse administrators with the challenge of properly orienting these nurses to the individual healthcare facility, the U.S. healthcare system, and the scope and standards of professional nursing practice. Increasing international staff can address improving cultural competence of all staff. However, employing such a solution to this country's nursing shortage is at the expense of the originating country and its population, and thus may pose a significant ethical concern for the nurse administrator.

Another continuing trend is the aging of the nursing workforce. As this demographic fact continues, nurse administrators must respond to the increasing needs of the aging employee by improving workplace satisfaction with accommodations in scheduling and the physical nursing environment, as well as provision of specific benefits, including affordable health insurance, elder-parent care, college tuition plans for their own children, and retirement or pension benefits.

Older nurses will require more ergonomically effective ways of delivering care. Rapidly changing information technology, while useful in healthcare settings to prevent or reduce errors and decrease nurse time spent on paperwork, can present a challenge to older staff. At the same time, nurse administrators should push for a greater use of technology both in direct and indirect patient care settings as a means of improving efficiency, reducing costs, and enhancing effective communication and safety .

Blended levels of experience and education create a dynamic profession, as increasing numbers of nurses enter the field as second-degree program graduates. Many of these nurses bring with them an entirely different skill set from former careers, as well as different educational backgrounds and college-level education in a variety of fields. Along with the mix of education and experience, this creates intergenerational workforce diversity, as the age range of new graduate nurses is even more varied due to this second-career trend. Nurse administrators must be prepared to harness this variety of experience and talent, leverage expectations of the individuals, and create a harmonious blend among their nursing units or staff. The nurse administrators must also exhibit flexibility in assessing and adapting to the varying needs and expectations of this dynamic workforce through such initiatives as established formal orientation and coaching sessions and continuing education programs focused on appreciating personality differences, diversity of expectations, and communication mechanisms.

The rising cost of healthcare represents almost one-fifth of the U.S. gross domestic product. Without critical intervention, this trend will continue to rise. Nurse administrators should represent nursing in these discussions and advocate for population health goals as well as patient and family interests in these discussions. Reaffirming nursing's value in these efforts is critical as they advocate for solutions that increase access and reduce costs while improving the safety and quality of health care.

Natural and man-made disasters constitute major threats to the community at large, and healthcare institutions play a major role in pre-event planning, situational response, and post-disaster mitigation. Nurse administrators must engage in emergency planning, as well as make staff aware of and prepared for their roles during an emergency and provide them the resources and training to be prepared for those roles. Surge capacity, staff response, and emergency communications will be among the things the public will expect facilities and organizations to be prepared to handle in a disaster.

The movement in global society to reduce mankind's impact on our natural world is creating emphasis in healthcare sectors on limiting damages to the environment and to communities from medical waste. Initiatives have been formed within nursing to address this issue and promote environmentally sound practices in nursing. Nurses work to establish and maintain public awareness and support efforts to decrease the risks and effects of pollutants in the environment and contaminants and other hazardous materials found in consumer products. Nurse administrators should be prepared to include these considerations in their business decisions, and they should become vocal advocates for environmental and public health among their colleagues and communities.

As issues and trends evolve, nursing with its dynamism and flexibility is poised to serve as a catalyst for positive approaches to this evolution. Nurse administrators must have a keen sense of the need for change and react with courage, fortitude, and wisdom. The ability of nurses and nurse leaders to partner with healthcare consumers, interdisciplinary colleagues, the community, and other stakeholders to achieve a mutually beneficial outcome can provide the stability needed to weather the tempest of changing times.

Standards of Nursing Administration Practice

Function of Standards

The standards, which are comprised of the standards of practice (pages 25–33) and the standards of professional performance (pages 34–44), are authoritative statements by which nurses practicing within the role, population, and specialty governed by this document (*Nursing Administration: Scope and Standards of Practice*) and describe the duties that they are expected to competently perform. The standards published herein may be utilized as evidence of the legal standard of care governing nurses practicing within the role, population, and specialty governed by this document. The standards are subject to change with the dynamics of the nursing profession and as new patterns of professional practice are developed and accepted by the nursing profession and the public. In addition, specific conditions and clinical circumstances may also affect the application of the standards at a given time; such as during a natural disaster. The standards are subject to formal, periodic review and revision.

The measurement criteria that appear below each standard are not all-inclusive and do not establish the legal standard of care. Rather, the measurement criteria are specific, measurable elements that can be used by nursing professionals to measure professional performance. Nurses practicing within this particular role, population, and specialty can identify opportunities for development and improvement by evaluating performance on these elements.

STANDARDS OF PRACTICE

STANDARD 1. ASSESSMENT
The nurse administrator collects comprehensive data pertinent to the issue, situation, or trends.

Measurement Criteria:

The nurse administrator:

- Collects data in a systematic and ongoing process.

- Involves healthcare providers and other stakeholders, as appropriate, in holistic data collection related to context and environment.

- Prioritizes data collection activities based on immediate or anticipated needs.

- Uses appropriate evidence-based assessment techniques and instruments in collecting pertinent data.

- Uses analytical models and problem-solving tools.

- Identifies gaps and necessary mechanisms to address and resolve missing or insufficient data, information, and knowledge resources.

- Synthesizes available data, information, and knowledge relevant to the situation to identify patterns and variances.

- Documents relevant data in a retrievable format.

STANDARD 2. IDENTIFIES ISSUES, PROBLEMS, OR TRENDS
The nurse administrator analyzes the assessment data to determine the issues, problems, or trends.

Measurement Criteria:

The nurse administrator:

- Demonstrates the ability to examine and synthesize complex data, information, and knowledge representations.

- Promotes the integration of clinical, human resource, and financial data to support and enhance decision-making.

- Derives the issues, problems, or trends from assessment data.

- Validates the issues, problems, or trends with the healthcare providers and other stakeholders when possible and appropriate.

- Documents issues, problems, or trends in a manner that facilitates the determination of the plan and expected outcomes.

STANDARD 3. OUTCOMES IDENTIFICATION
The nurse administrator identifies expected outcomes for a plan individualized to the situation.

Measurement Criteria:

The nurse administrator:

- Involves healthcare providers and other stakeholders in formulating expected outcomes when possible and appropriate.

- Derives culturally appropriate expected outcomes from identification of the issues, problems, or trends.

- Defines expected outcomes in terms of values, ethical considerations, environment, or situation, considering associated risks, benefits and costs, and current scientific evidence.

- Includes a time estimate for attainment of expected outcomes.

- Develops expected outcomes that provide direction for continuity of care.

- Modifies expected outcomes based on changes in the status of the issue, problem, or trend, or evaluation of the situation.

- Documents expected outcomes as measurable goals.

STANDARD 4. PLANNING

The nurse administrator develops a plan that prescribes strategies and alternatives to attain expected outcomes.

Measurement Criteria:

The nurse administrator:

- Develops an individualized plan considering characteristics of the situation.

- Develops the plan and establishes the plan priorities in partnership with the appropriate stakeholders.

- Includes strategies within the plan that address each of the identified issues, problems, or trends.

- Incorporates an implementation pathway or timeline within the plan.

- Utilizes the plan to provide direction to members of the healthcare team and other stakeholders.

- Defines the plan to reflect current statutes, rules and regulations, and standards.

- Integrates current trends and research affecting care in the planning process.

- Considers the economic impact of the plan.

- Uses standardized language or recognized terminology to document the plan.

- Participates in the design and development of multidisciplinary and interdisciplinary processes to address the situation or issue.

- Contributes to the development and continuous improvement of organizational systems that support the planning process.

- Supports the integration of clinical, human, and financial resources to enhance and complete the decision-making processes.

STANDARD 5. IMPLEMENTATION
The nurse administrator implements the identified plan.

Measurement Criteria:

The nurse administrator:

- Implements the plan in a safe and timely manner.

- Documents implementation and any modifications, including changes or omissions, of the identified plan.

- Utilizes evidence-based interventions and treatments specific to the problem, issue, or diagnosis.

- Facilitates utilization of systems and community resources to implement the plan.

- Collaborates with nursing colleagues and others to implement the plan.

- Incorporates new knowledge and strategies to initiate change and achieve desired outcomes.

- Implements the plan using principles and concepts of project or systems management.

- Fosters organizational systems that support implementation of the plan.

STANDARD 5A: COORDINATION

The nurse administrator coordinates the implementation and other associated processes.

Measurement Criteria:

The nurse administrator:

- Coordinates implementation of the plan and the associated activities and efforts.

- Coordinates human, capital, system, and community resources and measures, including environmental modifications, necessary to implement the plan.

- Provides leadership in the coordination of multidisciplinary health-care resources for integrated delivery of care and services.

- Promotes communication systems for an open and transparent organization.

STANDARD 5B: HEALTH PROMOTION, HEALTH TEACHING, AND EDUCATION

The nurse administrator employs strategies to foster health promotion, health teaching, and the provision of other educational services and resources.

Measurement Criteria:

The nurse administrator:

- Contributes to the design, development, implementation, and evaluation of educational programs, including continuing education and other professional development programs, needed to implement the plan.

- Promotes the incorporation of materials, teaching methods, and other educational tools and services appropriate to the situation and the learner's developmental level, learning needs, readiness and ability to learn, language preference, health literacy, and cultural values and beliefs.

- Identifies the need to integrate learning resources into healthcare systems that address health content topics such as healthy lifestyles, risk-reducing behaviors, developmental needs, activities of daily living, and preventive self-care.

- Promotes awareness and education of the healthcare consumer with regard to appropriate data collection, information sharing, information access, and associated issues.

- Evaluates health information resources, such as the Internet, within the area of practice for accuracy, readability, and comprehensibility to help individuals, families, healthcare providers, and others access quality health information.

- Creates opportunities for feedback and evaluation of the effectiveness of the educational content and teaching strategies used for the continuing education and professional development programs necessary to implement the plan.

STANDARD 5C: CONSULTATION

The nurse administrator provides consultation to influence the identified plan, enhance the abilities of others, and effect change.

Measurement Criteria:

The nurse administrator:

- Synthesizes data, information, theoretical frameworks, and evidence when providing consultation.

- Facilitates the effectiveness of a consultation by involving the stakeholders in decision-making and negotiating role responsibilities.

- Communicates consultation recommendations that influence the identified plan, facilitate understanding by involved stakeholders, enhance the work of others, and effect change.

STANDARD 6. EVALUATION
The nurse administrator evaluates progress towards attainment of outcomes.

Measurement Criteria:

The nurse administrator:

- Conducts a systematic, ongoing, and criterion-based evaluation of the outcomes in relation to the structures and processes prescribed by the plan and the indicated timeline.

- Provides evaluation processes built on appropriate research methods, evaluation tools, and metrics.

- Includes the stakeholders involved in the care or situation in the evaluative process.

- Evaluates the effectiveness of the planned strategies in relation to nurse-sensitive indicators, stakeholder responses, and the attainment of the expected outcomes.

- Documents the results of the evaluation.

- Uses the results of the evaluation analyses to make or recommend process or structural changes including policy, procedure, or protocol documentation, as appropriate.

- Synthesizes the results of the evaluation analyses to determine the impact of the plan on the affected patients, families, groups, communities, populations, and institutions, networks, and organizations.

- Disseminates the results to the stakeholders involved in the care or situation, as appropriate, in accordance with state and federal laws and regulations.

STANDARDS OF PROFESSIONAL PERFORMANCE

STANDARD 7. QUALITY OF PRACTICE
The nurse administrator systematically enhances the quality and effectiveness of nursing practice, nursing services administration, and the delivery of services.

Measurement Criteria:

The nurse administrator:

- Uses creativity and innovation in nursing practice to improve care delivery and population outcomes.

- Implements initiatives to evaluate the need for change.

- Drives quality improvement programs and activities.

- Uses the results of quality improvement activities to initiate changes in nursing practice and in the healthcare delivery system.

- Incorporates new knowledge to initiate changes in nursing practice to achieve desired outcomes.

- Assures the presence of effective mechanisms for the development, implementation, and evaluation of policies, procedures, standards, and guidelines.

- Assures the development and implementation of an effective, ongoing program to measure, assess, and improve the quality of care, treatment, and services delivered.

- Evaluates the practice environment and quality of nursing care rendered in relation to existing evidence, identifying opportunities for the generation and use of research.

- Participates in the evaluation and regulation of individuals as appropriate through privileging, credentialing, or certification processes.

- Demonstrates quality by documenting the application of the nursing process in a responsible, accountable, and ethical manner.

- Adheres to applicable professional standards and regulations.

- Obtains and maintains professional certification if eligible.

STANDARD 8. EDUCATION
The nurse administrator attains knowledge and competency that reflects current practice.

Measurement Criteria:

The nurse administrator:

- Participates in ongoing educational activities related to appropriate knowledge bases and professional issues.

- Demonstrates a commitment to lifelong learning through self-reflection and inquiry to identify learning needs.

- Seeks experiences and independent learning activities that reflect current practice in order to develop, maintain, and improve skills and competence in the nurse administrator role.

- Acquires knowledge and skills appropriate to the specialty area, practice setting, role, or situation.

- Maintains professional records that provide evidence of competency and lifelong learning.

- Uses current research findings and other evidence to enhance role performance and increase knowledge of professional issues.

STANDARD 9. PROFESSIONAL PRACTICE EVALUATION

The nurse administrator evaluates own nursing practice in relation to professional practice standards and guidelines, relevant statutes, rules, and regulations.

Measurement Criteria:

The nurse administrator:

- Applies knowledge of current practice standards, guidelines, statutes, rules, and regulations in practice.

- Demonstrates respect for diversity in all interactions as reflected in such behaviors as cultural, ethnic, and generational sensitivity.

- Engages in self-evaluation of practice on a regular basis, identifying areas of strength as well as areas in which professional development would be beneficial.

- Obtains informal and formal feedback regarding role performance from professional colleagues, representatives and administrators of corporate entities, and others.

- Participates in systematic peer review of others as appropriate.

- Interacts with peers and colleagues to enhance own professional nursing practice and role performance.

- Takes action to achieve goals identified during the evaluation process.

- Provides rationales for practice beliefs, decisions, and actions as part of the informal and formal evaluation processes.

STANDARD 10. COLLEGIALITY

The nurse administrator interacts with and contributes to the professional development of peers and colleagues.

Measurement Criteria:

The nurse administrator:

- Shares knowledge and skills with peers and colleagues as evidenced by such activities as care conferences or presentations at formal or informal meetings.

- Provides peers with feedback regarding their practice and role performance.

- Maintains empathetic and caring relationships with peers and colleagues.

- Establishes an environment that is conducive to the education of healthcare professionals.

- Assures the presence of a supportive and healthy work environment.

- Models expert practice to interdisciplinary team members and healthcare consumers.

- Assists staff in developing and maintaining competency in the analytic process.

- Mentors other registered nurses, nurse administrators, and colleagues as appropriate.

- Participates on multi-professional teams that contribute to role development and, directly or indirectly, advance nursing practice and health services.

STANDARD 11. COLLABORATION

The nurse administrator collaborates with all levels of nursing staff, interdisciplinary teams, executive leaders, and other stakeholders.

Measurement Criteria:

The nurse administrator:

- Communicates with healthcare providers and other stakeholders regarding care and services and the nurse's role in the provision of care.

- Collaborates in creating a documented plan focused on outcomes and decisions related to care and delivery of services.

- Partners with others to enhance health care and employee satisfaction through interdisciplinary activities such as education, consultation, management, technological development, or research opportunities.

- Models an interdisciplinary process with other members of the healthcare team.

- Documents plans, communications, rationales for plan changes, and collaborative discussions.

STANDARD 12. ETHICS

The nurse administrator integrates ethical provisions in all areas of practice.

Measurement Criteria:

The nurse administrator:

- Incorporates *Code of Ethics for Nurses with Interpretive Statements* (ANA, 2001) to guide practice.

- Assures the preservation and protection of the autonomy, dignity, and rights of individuals.

- Maintains confidentiality within legal and regulatory parameters.

- Assures a process to identify and address ethical issues within nursing and the organization.

- Participates on multidisciplinary and interdisciplinary teams that address ethical risks, benefits, and outcomes.

- Informs administrators or others of the risks, benefits, and outcomes of programs and decisions that affect healthcare delivery.

- Demonstrates a commitment to practicing self-care, managing stress, and connecting with self and others.

STANDARD 13. RESEARCH
The nurse administrator integrates research findings into practice.

Measurement Criteria:

The nurse administrator:

- Utilizes the best available evidence, including research findings, to guide practice decisions.

- Creates a supportive environment with sufficient resources for nursing research, scholarly inquiry, and the generation of knowledge.

- Assures research priorities align with the organization's strategic plans and objectives and include an appropriate nursing focus.

- Formally disseminates research findings through activities such as presentations, publications, and consultation.

STANDARD 14. RESOURCE UTILIZATION

The nurse administrator considers factors related to safety, effectiveness, cost, and impact on practice in the planning and delivery of nursing and other services.

Measurement Criteria:

The nurse administrator:

- Evaluates factors such as safety, effectiveness, availability, cost and benefits, efficiencies, and impact on practice when choosing practice options that would result in the same expected outcome.

- Develops innovative solutions that address effective resource utilization and maintenance of quality.

- Assures that resource allocations are based on identified needs and valid nursing workload measures.

- Secures organizational resources to create a work environment conducive to completing the identified plan and conducting the critical assessment and evaluation of desired outcomes.

- Develops evaluation strategies to demonstrate cost effectiveness, cost benefit, environmental impact, and efficiency factors associated with nursing practice.

- Develops evaluation methods to measure safety and effectiveness for interventions and outcomes.

- Promotes the value of the intellectual capital of the organization and appropriate measures to develop and expand this resource.

- Establishes strategies and mechanisms to promote organizational acceptance of appropriate roles for the utilization of all staff.

- Optimizes fiscal resource allocation to support current and potential objectives and initiatives.

- Leads in promoting the appropriate use of innovative applications and new technologies, including consideration of the impact on global environmental health and sustainability.

- Promotes activities that assist others, as appropriate, in becoming informed about costs, risks, and benefits of plans and solutions.

STANDARD 15. LEADERSHIP
The nurse administrator provides leadership in the professional practice setting and the profession.

Measurement Criteria:

The nurse administrator:

- Engages in teamwork as a team player and a team builder.

- Works to create and maintain healthy work environments in local, regional, national, or international communities.

- Displays the ability to define a clear vision, the associated goals, and a plan to implement and measure progress.

- Exhibits creativity and flexibility through times of change.

- Demonstrates energy, excitement, and a passion for quality work.

- Willingly accepts mistakes by self and others, thereby creating a culture in which risk-taking is not only safe, but expected.

- Inspires loyalty through valuing of people as the most precious asset in an organization.

- Serves in key roles in the work setting by participating on committees, councils, and administrative teams.

- Promotes advancement of the profession through participation in professional organizations.

- Influences decision-making bodies to improve patient care, health services, and policies.

- Provides direction to enhance the effectiveness of the multidisciplinary or interdisciplinary team.

- Assures that protocols or guidelines reflect evidence-based practice, include accepted changes in care management, and address emerging problems.

- Promotes communication of information and advancement of the profession through writing, publishing, and presentations for professional or lay audiences.

- Designs innovations to effect change in practice and outcomes.

STANDARD 16. ADVOCACY

The nurse administrator advocates for the protections and rights of individuals, families, communities, populations, healthcare providers, nursing and other professions, and institutions and organizations, especially related to health and safety.

Measurement Criteria:

The nurse administrator:

- Supports the involvement of individuals in their own care.

- Supports access by individuals to their own personal health information and development of awareness of how that information may be used and accessed by others.

- Supports the individual's right and ability to supplement, request correction of, and share their personal health data and information.

- Evaluates factors related to privacy, security, and confidentiality in the use and handling of health information.

- Integrates advocacy into the design, implementation, and evaluation of policies, programs and services, and systems.

- Demonstrates skill in advocating before providers, public representatives and decision-makers, and other stakeholders.

- Exhibits fiscal responsibility and integrity in policy development and advocacy activities and processes.

- Strives to resolve conflicting expectations from populations, providers, and other stakeholders to promote safety, guard their best interests, and to preserve the professional integrity of the nurse.

- Serves as an expert for peers, populations, providers, and other stakeholders in promoting and implementing health policies.

REFERENCES

American Nurses Association (1991). *Standards for organized nursing services and responsibilities of nurse administrators across all settings.* Kansas City, MO: Author.

American Nurses Association (1995). *Scope and standards for nurse administrators.* Washington, DC: American Nurses Publishing.

American Nurses Association (2001). *Code of ethics for nurses with interpretive statements.* Washington, DC: Author.

American Nurses Association (2002). *Nursing's agenda for the future: A call to the nation.* Washington, DC: Author.

American Nurses Association (2004). *Scope and standards for nurse administrators, 2nd edition.* Washington, DC: Nursesbooks.org.

American Nurses Credentialing Center (2008). *Application Manual Magnet Recognition Program®.* Silver Spring, MD: Author.

American Organization of Nurse Executives (2005). AONE nurse executive competencies. *Nurse Leader,* February, 50-6. Retrieved on February 18, 2009, from http://www.aone.org/aone/pdf/February%20Nurse%20Leader—final%20draft—for%20web.pdf

Asiton, M., & Chou, D. (2005). Just culture and strong interventions at the point of care. *Point of Care, 4* (4), 154–157.

Burns, J.M. (1978). *Leadership.* New York: Harper and Row.

Carroll, T. (2005). Leadership skills and attributes of women and nurse executives: Challenges for the 21st century. Nursing Administration Quarterly, 29 (2), 146–153.

Curtin, L. (2007). The perfect storm: Managed care, aging adults, and a nursing shortage. Nursing Administration Quarterly, 31 (2), 105–114.

Greenleaf, R. K. (1978). *Servant: Leader and follower.* New York: Paulist Press.

Havens, D.S., Wood, S.O., & Leeman, J. (2006). Improving nursing practice and patient care: Building capacity with appreciative inquiry. *Journal of Nursing Administration, 36* (10), 463–470.

Institute of Medicine (1999). *To err is human: Building a safer health system.* Washington, DC: National Academies Press.

Institute of Medicine (2003). *Keeping patients safe: Transforming the work environment of nurses.* Washington, DC: National Academies Press.

Institute of Medicine (2003). *Patient safety: Achieving a new standard of care.* Washington, DC: National Academies Press.

Neill, M.W., & Saunders, N.S. (2008). Servant leadership: Enhancing quality of care and staff satisfaction. *The Journal of Nursing Administration, 38* (9), 395–399.

Rearick, E. (2007). Enhancing success in transition service coordinators: Use of transformational leadership. *Professional Case Management, 12* (5), 283–287.

Robbins, B., & Davidhizar, R. (2007). Transformational leadership in health-care today. *The Health Care Manager, 26* (3), 234–239.

Weston, M.J. (2008). Defining control over nursing practice and autonomy. *The Journal of Nursing Administration, 38* (9) 404–408.

Appendix A.
ANA Bill of Rights for Registered Nurses (2001)

Registered nurses promote and restore health, prevent illness, and protect the people entrusted to their care. They work to alleviate the suffering experienced by individuals, families, groups and communities. In so doing, nurses provide services that maintain respect for human dignity and embrace the uniqueness of each patient and the nature of his or her health problems, without restriction with regard to social or economic status. To maximize the contributions nurses make to society, it is necessary to protect the dignity and autonomy of nurses in the workplace. To that end, the following rights must be afforded:

1. Nurses have the right to practice in a manner that fulfills their obligations to society and to those who receive nursing care.

2. Nurses have the right to practice in environments that allow them to act in accordance with professional standards and legally authorized scopes of practice.

3. Nurses have the right to a work environment that supports and facilitates ethical practice, in accordance with the *Code of Ethics for Nurses with Interpretive Statements.*

4. Nurses have the right to freely and openly advocate for themselves and their patients, without fear of retribution.

5. Nurses have the right to fair compensation for their work, consistent with their knowledge, experience and professional responsibilities.

6. Nurses have the right to a work environment that is safe for themselves and for their patients.

7. Nurses have the right to negotiate the conditions of their employment, either as individuals or collectively, in all practice settings.

Adopted by the ANA, Board of Directors, June 26, 2001. © 2001 American Nurses Association.

APPENDIX B.
SCOPE AND STANDARDS FOR NURSE ADMINISTRATORS, SECOND EDITION (2004)

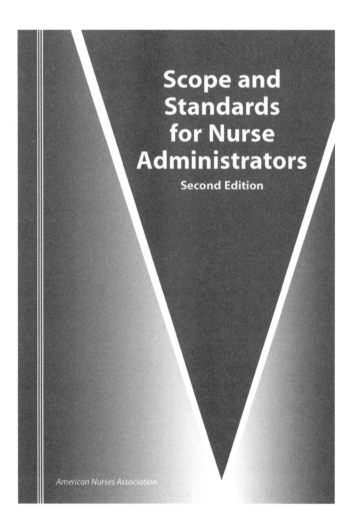

This appendix is not current and is of historical significance only.

Scope and Standards
for
Nurse Administrators
Second Edition

AMERICAN NURSES ASSOCIATION

nurses
books
.org

The Publishing Program of ANA

Washington, D.C.
2004

This appendix is not current and is of historical significance only.

Library of Congress Cataloging-in-Publication data

American Nurses Association.
  Scope and standards for nurse administrators / American Nurses
Association.-- 2nd ed.
      p. ; cm.
Includes bibliographical references and index.
  ISBN 1-55810-217-5
  1. Nursing services--Administration--Standards--United States. 2. Nurse
administrators--United States.
    [DNLM: 1. Nursing Services--standards--United States. 2. Nurse
Administrators--standards--United States. WY 100 A512sb 2003] I. Title.

  RT89.A448 2003
  362.17'3'068--dc22
                              2003023833

Disclaimer: The American Nurses Association (ANA) is a national professional association. This ANA publication—*Scope and Standards of Practice for Nurse Administrators, Second Edition*—reflects the thinking of the nursing profession on various issues and should be reviewed in conjunction with state board of nursing policies and practices. State law, rules, and regulations govern the practice of nursing, while *Scope and Standards of Practice for Nurse Administrators, Second Edition* guides nurses in the application of their professional skills and responsibilities.

Published by nursesbooks.org
The Publishing Program of ANA

American Nurses Association
600 Maryland Avenue, SW
Suite 100 West
Washington, DC 20024
1-800-274-4ANA
http://www.nursingworld.org/

© 2004 American Nurses Association. All rights reserved. No part of this book may be reproduced or utilized in any form or any means, electronic or mechanical, including photocopying and recording, or by any information storage and retrieval system, without permission in writing from the publisher.

ISBN 1-55810-217-5

03SSNA   10M   12/03

This appendix is not current and is of historical significance only.

CONTENTS

This appendix is not current and is of historical significance only.

—— = Not included in this reproduction.*

PREFACE

This document reflects the significant thinking, dialogue, and consensus decision-making of the American Nurses Association (ANA) specially convened expert workgroup composed of nurse administrators from diverse work and organizational settings. The nurse administrators included recognized leaders in the specialty. Each maintains membership in one or more specialty nursing organizations or other professional affiliations such as the American Organization of Nurse Executives (AONE), Association of State and Territorial Directors of Nursing (ASTDN), Hospice and Palliative Nurses Association (HPNA), and American Nurses Credentialing Center (ANCC) Magnet Recognition hospitals.

As part of the scope and standards development process, the workgroup examined previous versions of the ANA scope and standards of practice for nurse administrators (ANA, 1991, 1995), other associated standards documents (ANCC, 2003; ANA, 2004, 2000, 1996), and numerous contemporary and historical resources (AACN, 2002; AHCA, 2002; AHA, 2002, 2001; ANA, 2003, 2001, 1998; McClure & Langshawe, 2002; U.S. HHS, 2002). The 18-month process relied solely on telephone and electronic mail communication technologies. Upon completion of a draft document, the workgroup sought national and international comments during the field review period and posting at www.Nursingworld.org. This publication is the product of the workgroup's careful review and incorporation of those comments, review by the ANA Committee on Nursing Practice Standards and Guidelines, and final review and approval by the Congress on Nursing Practice and Economics.

CONTRIBUTORS

Workgroup:

Mary Etta Mills, ScD, RN, CNAA, FAAN, Chair
Barbara L. Baylis, MSN, RN, CPHQ
Doreen K. Frusti, MSN, MS, RN
Ada Sue Hinshaw, PhD, RN, FAAN
Patricia M. Kelley, RN, CHPN
Candia Baker Laughlin, MS,RN,C
Judy Lentz, RN, MSN, OCN, NHA
Joy F. Reed, EdD, RN
Karen Rush, BSN, BSW, CHPN
Jane Wall, RN, MSN, CNA

ANA Staff

Office of Nursing Practice & Policy
Carol Bickford, PhD, RN
Mary Jean Schumann, MSN, RN, MBA CPNP
Yvonne Hulme, BBA

STANDARDS FOR NURSE ADMINISTRATORS

Standards of Practice

STANDARD 1. ASSESSMENT
The nurse administrator develops, maintains, and evaluates patient and staff data collection systems and processes to support the practice of nursing and delivery of patient/client/resident care.

STANDARD 2. PROBLEMS/DIAGNOSIS
The nurse administrator develops, maintains, and evaluates an environment that empowers and supports the professional nurse in analysis of assessment data and in decisions to determine relevant problems and diagnoses.

STANDARD 3. IDENTIFICATION OF OUTCOMES
The nurse administrator develops, maintains, and evaluates information systems and processes that promote desired, patient/client/resident-defined, professional, and organizational outcomes.

STANDARD 4. PLANNING
The nurse administrator develops, maintains, and evaluates organizational systems to facilitate planning for the delivery of care.

STANDARD 5. IMPLEMENTATION
The nurse administrator develops, maintains, and evaluates organizational systems that support implementation of plans and delivery of care across the continuum.

STANDARD 6. EVALUATION
The nurse administrator evaluates the plan and its progress in relation to the attainment of outcomes.

Standards of Professional Performance

STANDARD 7. QUALITY OF CARE AND ADMINISTRATIVE PRACTICE
The nurse administrator systematically evaluates the quality and effectiveness of nursing practice and nursing services administration.

STANDARD 8. PERFORMANCE APPRAISAL
The nurse administrator evaluates personal performance based on professional practice standards, relevant statutes, rules and regulations, and organizational criteria.

STANDARD 9. PROFESSIONAL KNOWLEDGE
The nurse administrator maintains and demonstrates current knowledge in the administration of healthcare organizations to advance nursing practice and the provision of quality healthcare services.

STANDARD 10. PROFESSIONAL ENVIRONMENT
The nurse administrator is accountable for providing a professional environment.

STANDARD 11. ETHICS
The nurse administrator's decisions and actions are based on ethical principles.

STANDARDS 12. COLLABORATION
The nurse administrator collaborates with nursing staff at all levels, interdisciplinary teams, executive leaders, and other stakeholders.

STANDARD 13. RESEARCH
The nurse administrator supports research and its integration into nursing and the delivery of healthcare services.

STANDARD 14. RESOURCE UTILIZATION
The nurse administrator evaluates and administers the resources of nursing services.

This appendix is not current and is of historical significance only.

INTRODUCTION

Health care has always been a complex enterprise. Changing public expectations, regulations, resources, and service demands continue to challenge registered nurses and nurse administrators. Evolving technologies, reimbursement models, and consumer demands dictate shorter lengths of stay and other changes in treatment patterns. These issues, combined with an aging population, result in increasing patient acuity and larger volumes of patients moving from traditional acute care settings into ambulatory and long-term care environments. Nursing, itself composed of an aging workforce population, bears the brunt of such stressors throughout the healthcare delivery continuum.

The expectation for continuity of care across service delivery settings has gained momentum with consumers, payers, and providers as a means of increasing effectiveness and efficiency. Contracts, mergers, and partnerships are creating integrated delivery systems designed to foster coordination of care processes and services. This further emphasizes the need for nursing administration leadership capable of developing creative strategic plans to lead the healthcare system now and in the future. Innovative use of information technology, systems, and nursing research, and new fields of inquiry such as genetics and telehealth, offer opportunities to create practice environments not previously possible.

A time of great change and challenge is also a time of great opportunity for innovation. Legislative and regulatory constraints surround the management of human and material resources. As the demand for registered nurses intensifies and the supply declines, service-education partnerships offer increased strength in planning, marketing, educating, and mentoring a future nursing workforce. Nursing personnel and other healthcare discipline shortages also demand better explication and utilization of scopes of practice and interdisciplinary collaborative partnerships in delivering care and leading the organization. Increasing diversity of the patient population and the workforce makes it essential to support an inclusive environment and culture that creates synergy in systems and processes. These challenges further illustrate the interdependency of private and public health systems and complicate the role of the nurse administrator, thereby demanding skills in evaluation of complex systems and the development of collaborative solutions.

Systems-based issues abound. Concerns for confidentiality and security of patient health information have raised new legislative and technological issues in the transmission of information within and between healthcare settings and healthcare providers, including healthcare documentation access, monitoring, and interventions managed from a distance. Ethical considerations for new care opportunities offered by growth in clinical trial research and life-extending technological, genetic, and biologic interventions can generate multidisciplinary development of healthcare law and regulations, and related policies and procedures. The need for mass casualty readiness and emergency preparedness supports systems integration across the community of healthcare facilities, public health services, emergency response organizations, and government resources.

Also of concern are the continuing themes of resource allocation and revenue production that stem from increased competition, regulation, and cost while striving for excellence. These serve as an impetus for monitoring, evaluation, and performance improvement based on data that instructs both the business and practice of healthcare delivery. Effective and dynamic nurse administration leadership will ensure well-planned organizational structures, inclusive decision-making, creative and supportive personnel policies, professional models of care that promote excellent patient care services, collegial interdisciplinary relationships, and professional growth and development of nursing staff. The impact and effectiveness of such leadership will determine the future role of nursing in an evolving healthcare environment.

This appendix is not current and is of historical significance only.

SCOPE OF PRACTICE

The nurse administrator has most often been described as a registered nurse whose primary responsibility is the management of healthcare delivery services and who represents nursing services. Today's nurse administrator, however, is positioned at the vanguard of expanded roles and career opportunities resulting from a dynamic healthcare environment.

While traditional roles in all healthcare settings continue to offer career growth, new opportunities have also been created with the expansion of responsibilities for management of multiple patient/client/resident care services. At the corporate systems level of integrated care organizations, nurse administrators have opportunities to structure and plan nursing care systems across a continuum of services offered in multiple settings. These roles offer new challenges for nurse administrators to apply diverse skills in organizational analysis, strategic planning, financial and human resources management, and professional development.

Entrepreneurial opportunities have grown for nurse administrators interested in developing their own enterprises, such as community health services, assisted living, and adult day care. Expansion of clinical trials examining new therapeutic interventions has created a demand for individuals able to organize and manage complex regimens within and across research settings. Consultative roles require individuals prepared to apply advanced administrative knowledge and skill to settings that would benefit from new approaches to the management of healthcare services.

Diverse fields—such as quality of care evaluation, clinical and organizational ethics, information management, and legal and regulatory oversight—increasingly demand well-prepared nurse administrators. Often the nurse administrator is the sole healthcare professional as expanding career opportunities set the stage for a broad scope of nursing administration practice, evolving beyond the familiar hospital-based healthcare delivery model.

Nursing administration occurs in a wide variety of settings. These include small facilities, integrated delivery systems, larger corporate-owned facilities, and organizational and academic settings, as well as ambulatory and nontraditional environments. How nurse administrator positions are made operational will depend upon the structure and complexity of the settings in which they occur. Nevertheless, nurse administrators at all levels and in all types of settings share a common set of standards to guide practice in achieving their goals.

Whatever the venue, the nurse administrator has the responsibility to create a work environment that facilitates and encourages nursing staff to demonstrate accountability for their own practice, an environment that empowers registered nurses at all levels of the organization to utilize critical thinking and participate in decision-making that affects nursing practice. Creating such an environment requires openness to entrepreneurial partnerships, interdisciplinary collaboration, and leadership by all nurse administrators.

Therefore, communication is critical and mandates that structures and processes facilitate both vertical and horizontal communication. Productivity, quality of care, and a safe and healthy workplace are all enhanced when concern for the individual seeking healthcare services is the top priority and when nursing administrators assure:

- adequate numbers of clinically competent staff,
- positive working relationships among the healthcare team,
- autonomy and accountability for nursing practice,
- nursing control of nursing practice and the practice environment,
- adequate compensation commensurate with responsibilities, education, and experience,
- access to education and research,
- access to appropriate technologies, and
- promotion of evidence-based practice.

Levels of Nursing Administration Practice

Nursing administration is conceptually divided into the administrative levels of the *nurse executive* and the *nurse manager*—each has a particular focus and makes a distinct contribution within a healthcare system. Some nurse administrator positions in diverse practice settings may contain components of more than one level. Individual nursing administrator positions may differ from the levels described in this scope of practice statement. However, most nursing administrative positions can be understood within this framework.

This appendix is not current and is of historical significance only.

Nurse Executive

The nurse executive is responsible and accountable for the overall management of nursing practice, nursing education and professional development, nursing research, nursing administration, and nursing services. The nurse executive holds the accountability to manage within the context of the organization as a whole, and to transform organizational values into daily operations yielding an efficient, effective, and caring organization. Such executive management responsibilities may by necessity be shared among many nurse administrators within the larger organization.

As the executive leader of a significant component of healthcare organization services and workforce, the nurse executive holds and exercises the authority to fulfill responsibilities to the profession, healthcare team, consumers of nursing services, and the organization. This authority is exercised globally across the organization's delivery systems and across the care continuum.

Serving as a catalyst and role model, the nurse executive provides leadership and direction in accord with the organization's mission and values and nursing's core ideology. The nurse executive collaborates with other professional disciplines to achieve organizational healthcare goals. The nurse executive is a partner with medicine, administrative executives, and other interdisciplinary organizational leaders to oversee practice and operations.

The nurse executive ensures the development, implementation, and evaluation of policies, programs, and services that are evidence-based and consistent with professional standards and values. The nurse executive is accountable for measurement, assessment, and improvement in nurse-sensitive patient and organizational outcomes, as well as the assurance of a professional nursing practice environment in which registered nurses are autonomous, govern their practice, and are empowered to provide effective, efficient, safe, and compassionate quality care. The practice environment is a critical factor in the recruitment and retention of registered nurses. The nurse executive is accountable to ensure the competence of registered nurses and their ongoing professional growth and development.

The nurse executive collaborates in the organization-wide healthcare delivery system and process design. Integral components of delivery system and process design include: the physical work environment (e.g., accommodating the aging worker), use of technology applications (i.e., more efficient, less personnel-intensive), nursing workload measurement based on patient need for nursing care, clinical and financial projection models, data collection and analysis, outcome identification and measurement, practice innovations, and recruitment and retention initiatives. Nurse executives provide leadership in professional, community, and legislative initiatives to shape the future of nursing, healthcare policy, and societal health.

The nurse executive addresses role accountabilities by collaborating with all relevant stakeholders to perform the following:

- Ensure that nursing practice is governed by professional nurses.

- Participate in the leadership of the healthcare organization as a full member of the executive team.

- Provide leadership in the strategic planning of the healthcare organization and nursing.

- Actively guide nursing as a profession to its objectives, such as those in *Nursing's Agenda for the Future* (ANA, 2002).

- Provide leadership in the determination of clinical, scholarly, and administrative nursing goals and directions, as well as the associated functions and processes necessary to achieve those goals.

- Acquire and allocate human, material, and financial resources for specific functions and processes.

- Evaluate and revise systems and processes of nursing services to ensure achievement of nurse-sensitive patient-, client-, or family-centered outcomes.

- Provide leadership in critical thinking, problem solving, managing conflict, and addressing ethical issues.

- Provide leadership in human resource development and management.

- Provide opportunities for consumer input into personal healthcare decisions and policy development.

- Ensure ongoing evaluation and innovation of services provided by nursing services and the organization as a whole.

- Facilitate the conduct, dissemination, and utilization of research to ensure evidence-based nursing, healthcare, management and administrative systems.

- Serve as a professional role model and mentor to motivate, develop, recruit, and retain future nurse administrators.

- Serve as an agent of change, assisting all staff in understanding the importance, necessity, impact, and process of change.

- Ensure that the diversity of the nursing workforce reflects population diversity.

- Ensure delivery of culturally-competent care.

- Support outcome measurement and evidence-based practice through participation in programs of study (e.g., National Database of Nursing Quality Indicators).

- Ensure measurement of patient/client/resident need for nursing care and then allocate resources accordingly.

- Ensure registered nurse participation in decision-making at varied levels of the organization.

- Ensure integration of appropriate technologies to meet the needs of professional nursing.

- Ensure a safe working environment.

- Strive to meet the Nursing Advisory Council on Nurse Education and Practice (NACNEP) goal of two-thirds of the registered nurse workforce prepared at the baccalaureate degree in nursing or higher education level by 2010.

In today's continuously evolving health care environment and delivery system models, the nurse executive may be identified by other titles such as the Chief Nursing Officer (CNO), Senior Vice President, Director of Clinical Nursing Services, Vice President for Patient Services, Service Chief, Chief Executive Officer, Chief Operating Officer, Director, President, Dean, or Associate Dean.

Nurse Manager

Nurse managers are responsible to a nurse executive and manage one or more defined areas of nursing services. Nurse managers advocate for and allocate available resources to promote efficient, effective, safe, and compassionate nursing care based on current standards of practice. They promote shared decision-making and professional autonomy by providing input—their own and that of their staff—into executive-level decisions, and by keeping staff informed of executive level activities and vice versa. Other responsibilities vary depending on the size and function of the organization.

Nurse managers coordinate activities between defined areas, and provide clinical and administrative leadership and expertise. They facilitate an atmosphere of interactive management and the development of collegial relationships among nursing personnel and others. They serve as a link between nursing personnel and other healthcare disciplines and workers throughout the organization and within the healthcare community. Nurse managers have major responsibility for the implementation of the vision, mission, philosophy, core values, evidence-based practice, and standards of the organization, and nursing services within their defined areas of responsibility.

Nurse managers are accountable for the environment in which clinical nursing is practiced. The nurse manager must create a learning environment that is open and respectful, and promotes the sharing of expertise to promote the benefits of health outcomes. The ability of nurse managers to enhance the practice environment is critical to the recruitment and retention of registered nurses with diverse backgrounds and appropriate education and experience. Nurse managers contribute to the strategic planning process, day-to-day operations, standards of care, and attainment of goals of the organization. Nurse managers collaborate with the nurse executive and others in organizational planning, innovation, and evaluation. In larger organizations, the nurse manager may include further delineated levels.

To fulfill the responsibilities described above, the nurse manager, in collaboration with nursing personnel and members of other disciplines, performs the following:

- Ensure that care is delivered with respect for individuals' rights and preferences.

- Participate in nursing and organizational policy formulation and decision-making involving staff.

- Accept organizational accountability for services provided to recipients.

- Evaluate the quality and appropriateness of health care.

- Coordinate nursing care with other healthcare disciplines, and assist in integrating services across the continuum of health care.

- Participate in the recruitment, selection, and retention of personnel, including staff representative of the population diversity.

- Assess the impact of, and plan strategies to address, such issues as:
  - Ethnic, cultural and diversity changes in the population
  - Political and social influences
  - Financial and economic issues
  - The aging of society and demographic trends
  - Ethical issues related to health care

- Assume responsibility for staffing and scheduling personnel. Assignments reflect appropriate utilization of personnel, considering scope of practice, competencies, patient/client/resident needs, and complexity of care.

- Ensure appropriate orientation, education, credentialing, and continuing professional development for personnel.

- Provide guidance for and supervision of personnel accountable to the nurse manager.

- Evaluate performance of personnel.

- Develop, implement, monitor, and be accountable for the budget for the defined area(s) of responsibility.

- Ensure evidence-based practice by participating in and involving the nursing staff in evaluative research activities.

- Provide or facilitate educational experiences for nursing and other students.

- Ensure shared accountability for professional practice.

- Advocate for a work environment that minimizes work-related illness and injury.

Like the nurse executive level, nurse administrators at the manager level may be identified by other titles, such as District Supervisor, Head Nurse, Department Head, Shift Manager, Clinical Coordinator, Project Manager, or Division Officer.

Qualifications of Nurse Administrators

Given the expectations of leadership and accountability of the nurse administrator, it is important to define the licensure, education, and experience required. Both the nurse executive and the nurse manager must hold an active registered nurse license and meet the requirements in the state in which they practice.

The nurse executive should hold a bachelor's degree and master's degree with a major in nursing. A doctoral degree in a relevant field is recommended, as is a nationally recognized certification in nursing administration.

The nurse manager should be prepared with a minimum of a bachelor's degree with a major in nursing. A master's degree with a focus in nursing is recommended, as is nationally recognized certification in nursing administration and an appropriate specialty.

The experience backgrounds of professional nurses who serve as nurse administrators must include clinical and administrative practice, which enables these registered nurses to consistently fulfill the responsibilities inherent in their respective administrative roles. The nurse administrator's practice draws on knowledge and research from such areas as noted in Table 1:

Table 1. Knowledge Base of Nurse Administrator Practice

• Care management systems	• Negotiation and conflict resolution
• Clinical practice guidelines and best practices	• Nursing research and other scholarly activities
• Consumer healthcare issues	• Organizational behavior and development
• Customer service	• Patient and employee safety regulations
• Data management	• Performance improvement
• Evidence-based nursing administration	• Practice innovation
• Fiscal management and financial outcome	• Professional nursing practice
• Health and public policy	• Professional practice environment
• Healthcare economics	• Standards of clinical nursing practice
• Healthcare evaluation and outcome measures	• Strategic visioning and planning
• Law, regulation, and ethics	• Systems for patient safety
• Management systems, processes, and analysis	• Technologies
• Marketing initiatives	• Trends in business practices
• Measurement of patient needs, outcomes, nursing workload	

Adapted from (VHA, 2000).

Summary of Nurse Executive and Nurse Manager

Table 2 compares the nurse administrator levels of nurse executive and nurse manager. Although some holding these positions have yet to complete the recommended educational and certification qualifications, this publication encourages all nurse administrators to achieve these professional milestones.

Table 2. Comparison of Qualifications and Responsibilities for Nurse Executive and Nurse Manager

Item	Nurse Executive	Nurse Manager
License	In state of practice	In state of practice
Education	BS, MS with focus in nursing Doctorate recommended	BS with focus in nursing MS with focus in nursing recommended
Certification	Nursing Administration recommended	Nursing Administration and appropriate specialty recommended
Authority	Organization-wide	One or more assigned areas
Area(s) of responsibility	Whole organization	Assigned areas only
Fiduciary responsibility	Input into system-wide budget planning Clinical/financial projections and budget for entire nursing department	Budget for assigned areas only
Specific responsibilities	Partner with other disciplinesand leaders Acquires resources for function and process Ensures development of policies, programs, and evidence-based practice consistent with standards Leads and directs patient care delivery systems Provides leadership in human resources development and management Visionary, strategic planner, change agent, practice innovator Accountable for continuous quality improvement for entire nursing system Assures nurse participation in decision-making	Direct supervision of assigned staff and interdisciplinary collaboration Manages recruitment, selection, retention, staffing, scheduling, and assigning Empowers staff to develop policies with management oversight Accepts organizational accountability for services provided Directs and manages personnel for assigned areas Implements the vision, mission, philosophy, core values, evidence-based practice, and standards in assigned areas Evaluates quality and appropriateness of healthcare delivery for assigned areas Empowers staff to participate in decision-making

This appendix is not current and is of historical significance only.

STANDARDS OF PRACTICE

AND

PROFESSIONAL PERFORMANCE

Standards are authoritative statements by which the nursing profession describes the responsibilities for which its practitioners are accountable. Consequently, standards reflect the values and priorities of the profession. Standards provide direction for professional nursing practice and a framework for the evaluation of this practice. Written in measurable terms, standards also define the nursing profession's accountability to the public and the outcomes for which registered nurses are responsible.

Specific measurement criteria accompany each of the standards of practice and professional performance for nurse administrators. At this time, research and the existing body of knowledge have not identified measurement criteria specific to either the nurse executive or nurse manager levels. Because the focus of this specialty practice tends to be on the development, implementation, and evaluation of the supporting framework, processes, and environment of nursing practice, the language of some of the standards and measurement criteria have been modified from those referenced in *Standards of Clinical Nursing Practice, 2nd Edition* (ANA, 1998). For example, the Standards of Practice describe the nursing process in nursing administration as assessment, problem/diagnosis, identification of outcomes, planning, implementation, and evaluation.

This appendix is not current and is of historical significance only.

STANDARDS OF PRACTICE

STANDARD 1. ASSESSMENT

The nurse administrator develops, maintains, and evaluates patient/ client/resident and staff data collection systems and processes to support the practice of nursing and delivery of patient/client/resident care.

Measurement Criteria

The nurse administrator:

1. Identifies assessment elements specific to nursing patient/client/resident indicators appropriate to a given organization.

2. Utilizes current research findings and current practice guidelines and standards to modify and improve data collection elements.

3. Monitors and evaluates assessment processes that are sensitive to the unique and diverse needs of individuals and target populations.

4. Identifies and documents the necessary resources to support data collection, and secures appropriate resources.

5. Analyzes the workflow related to effectiveness and efficiency of assessment processes.

6. Provides for efficient data collection as part of the institutional data collection systems.

7. Promotes, maintains, and evaluates a data collection system that has an accessible and retrievable format.

8. Initiates mechanisms to modify information systems and processes as needed to meet changing data requirements and needs.

9. Collaborates with appropriate departments to utilize assessment data to improve the operation of the healthcare environment and facility.

10. Evaluates assessment practices to assure timely, reliable, valid, and comprehensive data collection.

11. Facilitates integration of uniform assessment processes developed in collaboration with other healthcare disciplines across the continuum of care and internal and external to the organization.

12. Develops criteria and establishes procedures to assure confidentiality of data.

This appendix is not current and is of historical significance only.

STANDARD 2. PROBLEMS/DIAGNOSIS

The nurse administrator develops, maintains, and evaluates an environment that empowers and supports the professional nurse in analysis of assessment data and in decisions to determine relevant problems and diagnoses.

Measurement Criteria

The nurse administrator:

1. Identifies and secures adequate resources for decision analysis in collaboration with appropriate departments.

2. Assists and supports staff in developing and maintaining problem/diagnosis competency.

3. Facilitates interdisciplinary collaboration in data analysis and decision-making process.

4. Promotes an organizational climate that supports validation of problems/diagnoses.

5. Assures a system of documentation of problems/diagnoses that facilitates development of a patient/client/resident-centered plan of care and determination of desired outcomes.

6. Formulates a diagnosis of the organization's environment, culture, and priorities that direct and support care delivery.

STANDARD 3. IDENTIFICATION OF OUTCOMES

The nurse administrator develops, maintains, and evaluates information systems and processes that promote desired, patient/client/resident-defined, professional, and organizational outcomes.

Measurement Criteria

The nurse administrator:

1. Participates in the design and development of interdisciplinary processes to establish and maintain standards consistent with the identified outcomes.

2. Facilitates participation of registered nurses, other staff members, and patients/clients/residents in interdisciplinary identification of desired outcomes.

3. Assists in identification, development, and utilization of databases that include nursing measures and desired outcomes.

4. Facilitates registered nurse participation in the monitoring and evaluation of nursing care in accordance with established professional, regulatory, and organizational standards of practice.

5. Fosters establishment and continuous improvement of clinical guidelines related to outcomes that provide direction for continuity of care and that are attainable with available resources.

6. Collaborates with appropriate departments in the development of integrated systems to support nursing service delivery.

7. Promotes the integration of clinical, human resource, and financial data to support decision-making.

This appendix is not current and is of historical significance only.

STANDARD 4. PLANNING

The nurse administrator develops, maintains, and evaluates organizational systems to facilitate planning for the delivery of care.

Measurement Criteria

The nurse administrator:

1. Facilitates the development and continuous improvement of organizational systems in which plans related to the delivery of nursing services can be developed, modified, documented, and evaluated.

2. Facilitates the development and continuous improvement of organizational systems that promote plans and support the prioritization of activities related to patient/client/resident-directed care and the delivery of nursing services.

3. Facilitates the development and continuous improvement of mechanisms for plans to be recorded, reviewed, and updated across the continuum of care.

4. Promotes organizational processes that allow for creativity in the development of alternative plans for achieving desired, patient/client/resident-defined, cost-effective outcomes.

5. Fosters interdisciplinary planning and collaboration that focuses on the individuals and populations served.

6. Promotes the integration of applicable contemporary management and organizational theories, nursing and related research findings, and practice standards and guidelines into the planning process.

7. Assists and supports staff in developing and maintaining competency in the planning and change process.

8. Advocates for integration of policies into action plans for achieving desired outcomes.

9. Participates in the development, implementation, and use of a system to promote the rights and ethical treatment of the patient/client/resident and to ensure that abuse of the patient/client/resident's rights is reported.

10. Reviews and evaluates plans for appropriate utilization of staff at all levels of practice in accordance with the provisions of the state's nurse practice act and the professional standards of practice.

This appendix is not current and is of historical significance only.

11. Integrates clinical, human resource, and financial data to appropriately plan nursing and patient/client/resident care across a continuum.

12. Collaborates with appropriate departments and disciplines for the entire system to operate more efficiently in achieving outcomes.

13. Advocates for staff involvement in all levels of organizational planning and decision-making.

This appendix is not current and is of historical significance only.

STANDARD 5. IMPLEMENTATION

The nurse administrator develops, maintains, and evaluates organizational systems that support implementation of plans and delivery of care across the continuum.

Measurement Criteria

The nurse administrator:

1. Participates in the development, evaluation, and maintenance of organizational systems that integrate policies and procedures with regulations, practice standards, and clinical guidelines.

2. Designs and improves systems and identifies resources that support interventions that are consistent with the established plans.

3. Facilitates staff participation in decision-making regarding the development and implementation of organizational systems, and the specification of resources necessary for implementation of the plan.

4. Collaborates in the design and improvement of systems and the identification of resources that assure interventions are safe, effective, efficient, age-relevant, and culturally sensitive.

5. Collaborates in the design and improvement of systems and processes that assure interventions are implemented by the appropriate personnel.

6. Collaborates in the design and improvement of systems to assure appropriate and efficient documentation of interventions and patient/client/resident responses.

7. Leads initiatives in innovative programs and new implementation alternatives.

STANDARD 6. EVALUATION

The nurse administrator evaluates the plan and its progress in relation to the attainment of outcomes.

Measurement Criteria

The nurse administrator:

1. Promotes implementation of processes that deliver data and information to empower staff in decision-making.

2. Ensures educational opportunities for staff based on evaluation findings—specific to the population served, professional practice, available technologies, or required skills—to enhance quality in health care delivery.

3. Utilizes appropriate research methods and findings to evaluate and improve care processes, structures, and measurement of desired outcomes.

4. Facilitates the participation of staff in the systematic, interdisciplinary, and ongoing evaluation of programs, processes, and desired outcomes that promote organizational effectiveness.

5. Sets priorities for allocation of resources to conduct evaluative activities.

6. Ensures sufficient resources to provide for the critical assessment and evaluation of desired outcomes, including allocation of individual staff time for meaningful involvement.

7. Fosters participation and recognition of staff in internal and external, formal and informal organizational evaluation committees, teams, and task forces.

8. Advocates for and supports a process of participative decision-making.

9. Participates in the evaluation of all appropriate healthcare providers through privileging, credentialing, or certification processes.

10. Supports information handling processes and technologies to facilitate evaluation of effectiveness and efficiency of decisions, plans, and activities in relation to desired outcomes.

11. Promotes the development of policies, procedures, and guidelines based on research findings and institutional measurement of quality outcomes.

12. Utilizes data generated from outcomes research to develop innovative changes in care delivery.

This appendix is not current and is of historical significance only.

STANDARDS OF PROFESSIONAL PERFORMANCE

STANDARD 7. QUALITY OF CARE AND ADMINISTRATIVE PRACTICE

The nurse administrator systematically evaluates the quality and effectiveness of nursing practice and nursing services administration.

Measurement Criteria

The nurse administrator:

1. Leads the development, implementation, and improvement of care delivery models and services that meet or exceed customer expectations.

2. Identifies key indicators including measures of quality, safety, other outcomes of nursing practice, and customer needs and expectations.

3. Advocates for and participates in the development of clinical, operational, and financial processes from which key outcomes indicators can be derived, reported, and used for improvement.

4. Leads in creating and evaluating systems, processes and programs that support organizational and nursing core values and objectives.

5. Evaluates the care environment to ensure that it is safe and healthful for patients/client/resident and staff.

6. Implements performance improvement measures for the key indicators that have been identified.

This appendix is not current and is of historical significance only.

STANDARD 8. PERFORMANCE APPRAISAL

The nurse administrator evaluates personal performance based on professional practice standards, relevant statutes, rules and regulations, and organizational criteria.

Measurement Criteria

The nurse administrator:

1. Identifies industry trends and competencies in nursing administration and nursing practice, using a systematic process.

2. Engages in self-assessment of role accountabilities on a regular basis, identifying areas of strength as well as areas for professional and practice development.

3. Evaluates accomplishment of the strategic plan and the vision for professional nursing.

4. Seeks constructive feedback regarding one's own practice.

5. Takes action to achieve plans for performance improvement.

6. Participates in peer review as appropriate.

This appendix is not current and is of historical significance only.

STANDARD 9. PROFESSIONAL KNOWLEDGE

The nurse administrator maintains and demonstrates current knowledge in the administration of healthcare organizations to advance nursing practice and the provision of quality healthcare services.

Measurement Criteria

The nurse administrator:

1. Seeks experiences to advance one's skills and knowledge base in areas of responsibilities including the art and science of nursing, changes in healthcare systems, application of emerging technologies, and administrative practices.

2. Demonstrates a commitment to lifelong learning and ongoing professional development through such activities as education, certification, and participation in professional organizations.

3. Networks with state, regional, national, and global peers to share ideas and conduct mutual problem solving.

This appendix is not current and is of historical significance only.

STANDARD 10. PROFESSIONAL ENVIRONMENT

The nurse administrator is accountable for providing a professional environment.

Measurement Criteria

The nurse administrator:

1. Creates a professional practice environment that fosters excellence in nursing services.

2. Creates a climate of effective communication.

3. Fosters empowered decision-making, accountability, and autonomy in nursing practice for professional nurses.

4. Leads the organization of nursing services through a well-established nursing leadership structure, and is a formal authority participant in organizational leadership.

5. Establishes and promotes a framework for professional nursing practice built on core ideology which includes vision, mission, philosophy, core values, evidence-based practice, and standards of practice.

6. Assures the work environment is one of mutual respect for the individual and the profession.

7. Develops strategies to recruit and retain, mentor, assure quality education and training, and ensure meaningful work to maximize job satisfaction and professional development of nursing staff.

8. Promotes understanding and effective use of organization, management, and nursing theories and research.

9. Actively participates in the general and nursing management education and professional development of staff, students, and colleagues.

10. Advocates for organizational adherence to the ANA *Bill of Rights for Registered Nurses* (ANA, 2001a).

11. Shares knowledge and skills with students, colleagues and others, and acts as a role model and mentor.

This appendix is not current and is of historical significance only.

STANDARD 11. ETHICS

The nurse administrator's decisions and actions are based on ethical principles.

Measurement Criteria

The nurse administrator:

1. Advocates on behalf of recipients of services and personnel.

2. Maintains privacy, confidentiality, and security of patient/client/resident, staff, and organization data.

3. Adheres to the *Code of Ethics for Nurses with Interpretive Statements* (ANA, 2001b).

4. Assures compliance with regulatory and professional standards, as well as integrity in business practices.

5. Fosters a nondiscriminatory climate in which care is delivered in a manner sensitive to sociocultural diversity.

6. Assures a process to identify and address ethical issues within nursing and the organization.

This appendix is not current and is of historical significance only.

STANDARDS 12. COLLABORATION

The nurse administrator collaborates with nursing staff at all levels, interdisciplinary teams, executive leaders, and other stakeholders.

Measurement Criteria

The nurse administrator:

1. Facilitates and models collaboration within nursing services, the organization, and the community.

2. Collaborates with nursing staff and other disciplines at all levels in the development, implementation, and evaluation of programs and services.

3. Collaborates with administrative peers in determining the acquisition, allocation, and utilization of fiscal and human resources.

4. Develops and fosters relationships that support the continuous enhancement of care delivery and patient/client/resident and employee satisfaction.

This appendix is not current and is of historical significance only.

STANDARD **13. RESEARCH**

The nurse administrator supports research and its integration into nursing and the delivery of healthcare services.

Measurement Criteria

The nurse administrator:

1. Creates the environment and advocates for resources supportive of nursing research and scholarly inquiry.

2. Assures nursing research priorities align with nursing's and the organization's strategic plan and objectives.

3. Supports research that promotes evidence-based, clinically effective and efficient, nurse-sensitive patient/client/resident outcomes and other healthcare outcomes.

4. Facilitates the dissemination of research findings and the integration of evidence-based guidelines and practices into health care.

5. Supports procedures for review of proposed research studies, including protection of the rights of human subjects.

6. Identifies areas of clinical and administrative inquiry suitable for nurse researchers.

This appendix is not current and is of historical significance only.

Standard 14. Resource Utilization

The nurse administrator evaluates and administers the resources of nursing services.

Measurement Criteria

The nurse administrator:

1. Assures nursing workload is measured and resources are allocated based upon patient/client/resident need.

2. Develops systems to continuously monitor and measure the quality, safety, and outcomes of nursing services.

3. Develops, values, and expands the intellectual capital of the organization.

4. Assures and optimizes fiscal resource allocation to support current and potential nursing objectives and initiatives.

5. Provides fiscal oversight of allocated resources to optimize the provision of quality, cost-effective care.

6. Guides the delegation of responsibilities appropriate to the credentialing, education, and experience of staff.

7. Designs and negotiates organizational acceptance of appropriate roles for the utilization of all staff.

8. Monitors and evaluates appropriate utilization of staff.

9. Leads in promoting the appropriate use of innovative applications and new technologies throughout the continuum of care.

This appendix is not current and is of historical significance only.

GLOSSARY

Continuity of care. An interdisciplinary process that includes patients and significant others in the development and implementation of a plan of coordinated care. This process facilitates the transition of a patient/client/resident between settings and services, based on changing needs and available resources.

Core ideology. Vision, mission, philosophy, core values, evidence-based practice, and standards of practice.

Criteria. Relevant, measurable indicators of the standards of practice and professional performance.

Data collection systems and processes. Mechanisms and tools to identify and gather the necessary measures and information used in analysis, decision-making, action, and evaluation.

Evidence-based practice. A process based on the collection, interpretation, and integration of valid, important, and applicable data, information, and knowledge preferably derived from research findings to define the best approach or solution.

Healthcare organization. The total healthcare entity within which nursing services operate.

Intellectual capital. An organization's valued human knowledge, professional skills, applied experience, organizational technology, and customer relationships that provide its competitive edge in the industry or market.

Nurse administrator. A registered nurse whose primary responsibility is the management of healthcare services delivery, and who represents nursing services. For purposes of this document, the two levels of nurse administrators are those of the nurse executive and the nurse manager.

Nurse executive. A registered nurse who is accountable for nursing services, and manages from the perspective of the organization as a whole.

Nurse manager. A registered nurse who manages one or more defined areas within nursing services.

Nurse-sensitive. Reflective of the impact of nursing actions on patient/client/resident outcomes.

This appendix is not current and is of historical significance only.

Nursing services. The structure through which services, including direct care, education, or any other nursing related services, are provided by registered nurses and other personnel under the direction of a nurse administrator, within the scope of nursing practice, and in accordance with state laws and regulations.

Patient/client/resident. An individual, family, group, community, or population receiving care provided by nursing services.

Staff. All personnel reporting to the nurse administrator.

Standard. An authoritative statement defined, recognized, and published by the profession and by which the quality of practice, service, or education can be judged.

Standards of practice. Authoritative statements that describe a competent level of practice demonstrated through assessment, diagnosis and problem identification, identification of outcomes, planning, implementation, and evaluation.

Standards of professional performance. Authoritative statements that describe a competent level of behavior in the professional role, including activities related to quality of care and administrative practice, performance appraisal, education, professional environment, ethics, collaboration, research, and resource utilization.

This appendix is not current and is of historical significance only.

REFERENCES

American Association of Colleges of Nursing (2002). *Hallmarks of the professional nursing practice environment,* January. Washington, DC: AACN.

American Health Care Association (2002). *Competencies for senior nurse leaders in LTC vision statement. Washington, DC: AHCA.*

American Hospital Association (2001). *Workforce supply for hospitals and health systems: Issues and recommendations.* Washington, DC: AHA.

American Nurses Association. (2004). *Nursing: Scope and standards of practice.* Washington, DC: Nursesbooks.org.

American Hospital Association (2002). *In our hands: How hospital leaders can build a thriving workforce.* April. Chicago: AHA.

American Nurses Association. (2003). *Nursing's social policy statement, Second edition.* Washington, DC: Nursesbooks.org.

American Nurses Association (2002). *Nursing's agenda for the future: A call to the nation.* Washington, DC: ANA.

American Nurses Association (2001a). *Bill of rights for registered nurses.* Washington, DC: ANA.

American Nurses Association (2001b). *Code of ethics for nursing with interpretive statements.* Washington, DC: American Nurses Publishing.

American Nurses Association (2000). *Scope and standards of practice for nursing professional development.* Washington, DC: American Nurses Publishing.

American Nurses Association (1998). *Standards of clinical nursing practice, 2nd edition.* Washington, DC: American Nurses Publishing.

American Nurses Association. (1996). *Scope and standards of advanced practice registered nursing.* Washington, DC: American Nurses Publishing.

American Nurses Association (1995). *Scope and standards for nurse administrators.* Washington, DC: American Nurses Publishing.

American Nurses Association (1991). *Standards for organized nursing services and responsibilities of nurse administrators across all settings.* Kansas City, MO: ANA.

This appendix is not current and is of historical significance only.

American Nurses Credentialing Center 2003. *Magnet Recognition Program instruction and application process manual (2003–2004).* Washington, DC: ANCC.

McClure, M. & Hinshaw, A. S. (2002). *Magnet hospitals revisited: Attraction and retention of professional nurses.* Washington, DC: American Nurses Publishing.

VHA. National Nursing Leadership Council (2000). *Revolutionizing the future of nursing care: Defining the role of the chief nursing officer in the 21st century.* Irving, TX: VHA.

U.S. Department of Health and Human Services (2002). *The registered nurse population: Findings from the National Sample Survey of Registered Nurses, March 2000.* Washington, DC: Health Resources and Services Administration, Bureau of Health Professions, Division of Nursing.

INDEX

A

Abilities of nursing administrators, 19–20
Accountability, 4, 11, 17–20
  nurse executive and [2004], 60
  nurse manager and [2004], 63–64, 66
  professional environment and [2004],
    78
  [2004], 59
Advocacy
  authority and, 18
  for ethics, 10
  [2004], 79
  evaluation and, 33
  for nursing and health care, 2, 3, 22
  right of, 47
  for staff, 4, 9, 15
  standard of professional performance,
    44
  work environment and, 13, 18
  [2004], 62, 71, 72, 74, 75, 78, 81
Aging of nursing workforce, 2, 20, 22
  [2004], 56
American Nurses Association (ANA)
  Code of Ethics for Nurses with Interpretive
    Statements (2001), 10
  publications on nursing
    administration,
American Nurses Credentialing Center
  (ANCC), 9
American Organization of Nurse
  Executives (AONE), 13
Appreciative inquiry as practice
  framework, 7
Assessment
  evaluation and, 33
  standard of practice, 25
  [2004], 55
  [2004], 68
Association of State and Territorial
  Directors of Nursing (ASTDN)
  [2004], 54
Authority of nurse administrators
  (spheres of influence)

organization-wide, 12–15
program-focused, 18
project-based, 18–19
task-based, 18–19
unit-based/service-line, 15–18
Autonomy, 11
  Ethics and, 40
  Nurse manager and [2004], 62
  Professional environment and, 13
  [2004], 78
  See also Rights and responsibilities

B

Bill of Rights for Registered Nurses (2001),
  47
  See also Rights and responsibilities
Body of knowledge of nursing
  administration. *See* Knowledge
  base of nursing administration

C

Case management. *See* Coordination of
  care
Certification and credentialing, 11, 17,
  19, 35
  evaluation and [2004], 74
  nurse administrator and [2004], 74
  nurse executive and [2004], 64–66
  nurse manager and [2004], 64–66
  professional knowledge and [2004], 77
  resource utilization and [2004], 82
Client. *See* Patient
Code of Ethics for Nurses with Interpretive
  Statements (2001), 10. *See also* Ethics
Collaboration
  assessment and [2004], 68
  decision analysis [2004], 69
  defined [2004], 84
  nurse manager and [2004], 63
  planning and [2004], 71
  standard of professional performance,
    39
  [2004], 55, 80

Collegiality, 3, 16, 19
  standard of professional performance,
    38
  [2004], 57, 62
Communication
  importance of, 4, 7–8, 11–14
  [2004], 59, 78
Communities and nurse administrators,
    10, 12, 13, 23, 47
  advocacy and, 23, 24
  disaster response, 10, 23
  evaluation and, 33
  implementation and, 29
  [2004], 58, 60, 63, 80
Community and public health, 23
  [2004], 56, 57
Compensation, 11, 47
Competence and competencies
  collegiality and, 38
  education and, 36
  of nurse administrators, 3, 4, 21
  of staff, 15, 17, 58
  [2004], 60, 64, 69, 71
  See also Certification and credentialing
Confidentiality
  advocacy and, 44
  assessment and [2004], 68
  ethics and, 40
  [2004], 79
Conflicts of interest, 3
Consultation, 32
Continuity of care
  defined [2004], 83
  demand for [2004], 56
  outcome identification and, 27
  [2004], 70
Continuum of care, 4
  [2004], 68, 71, 82
Coordination of care, 30
Core ideology of nursing and nursing
    administration, 13
  [2004], 60, 78, 80
Credentialing. See Certification and
    credentialing
Criteria (measurement criteria)
  advocacy, 44

assessment, 25
  [2004], 68
collaboration, 39
  [2004], 80
collegiality, 38
consultation, 32
coordination, 30
defined [2004], 83
diagnosis [2004], 69
education, 31, 36
ethics, 40
  [2004], 79
evaluation, 33
  [2004], 74
implementation, 29
  [2004], 73
leadership, 43
outcome identification, 27
  [2004], 70
performance appraisal [2004], 76
planning, 28
  [2004], 71
professional environment [2004], 78
professional knowledge [2004], 77
professional practice evaluation, 37
quality of care and administrative
    practice [2004], 75
quality of practice, 35
  [2004], 55
research, 41
  [2004], 81
resource utilization, 42
  [2004], 82
trends, 26
Cultural competence, 20
Culture of quality and safety as practice
    framework, 6–7
  See also Quality entries; Safety
    assurance

D
Data and information analysis,
    synthesis, and use, 13, 21, 26, 32, 60
  confidentiality, ethics and, 68
  [2004], 79
  [2004], 69, 74

Marketing, 21
Measurement criteria. *See* Criteria
Mentoring, 2
  as practice framework, 7
Mission
  nurse executive and [2004], 60
  nurse manager and [2004], 63, 66
  professional environment and [2004],
    78
Multidisciplinary practice
  in coordination of care, 30
  ethics and, 40
  leadership and, 43
  in planning, 28
  See also Interdisciplinary practice

N
National Database of Nursing Quality
    Indicators [2004], 62
Nurse administrators
  abilities of, *19–20*
  advocacy and, 44
  assessment and, 25
  [2004], 55
  authority (spheres of influence), 12–
    19
  challenges, 2–3
  collaboration and, 39
  collegiality and, 38
  consultation and, 32
  coordination and, 30
  defined, 3
  [2004], 83
  education and, 19, 36
  ethics and, 10–11, 40
  evaluation and, 33
  frameworks for practice, 5–9
  health promotion, health teaching,
    and education, 31
  identifies issues, problems, or trends, 26
  [2004], 66
  implementation and, 29
  influence of, 12–19
  knowledge, skills, and abilities, 4, 9, 14,
    19–20
  leadership and, 2–3, 4, 43
  levels of practice [2004], 59–64

  nurse managers and executives and,
    ix, 12–13, 15–17, 19, 39
  organization-wide authority (sphere
    of influence), 12–15
  outcome identification, 27
  planning and, 28
  practice environments, 9–10
  professional practice evaluation, 37
  program-focused authority (sphere of
    influence), 18
  qualifications, 19–20
  [2004], 64–65
  quality of care and administrative
    practices, 35
  research, 42
  resource utilization and, 42
  responsibilities, 4
  roles, 3, 11
  skills of, 9–10
  unit-based/service-line authority
    (sphere of influence), 15–18
  and workforce, 7–8, 15, 18, 20
  See also Nurse executives; Nurse
    managers; Standards of practice;
    Standards of professional
    performance
Nurse executives
  defined [2004], 83
  nurse administrators and, *ix*, 12–13, 15,
    19, 39
  organization for (AONE), 13
  [2004], 59, 60–62, 65–66
Nurse managers
  defined [2004], 83
  nurse administrators and, *ix*, 12, 15, 16,
    17
  [2004], 59, 62–66
Nurse-sensitive (defined) [2004], 83
Nursing
  culture, 2, 6–7
  defined [2004], 84
  shortage, 2
  See also Education; Registered nurse (RN)
Nursing administration, 2
  See also Nurse administrators
Nursing Advisory Council on Nurse
    Education and Practice [2004], 62

Nursing process
  as practice framework, 6
  in nursing administration, 6, 13, 18
    [2004], 67
  in quality of practice, 35
  and standards of practice, 25
  See also Assessment; Diagnosis;
      Evaluation; Implementation;
      Outcomes identification; Planning
Nursing shortage, 20
Nursing workforce
  aging of, 2, 20, 22
  diversity of, 15,
  nurse administrators and, 7–8, 15, 18
  shortage of, 20
    [2004], 56, 60, 61, 62

O
Organization-wide authority (sphere of
    influence), 12–15
Organizational development resources,
    7
Outcomes identification, 60
  standard of practice, 27
    [2004], 55
    [2004], 70
Outcomes
  collaboration and, 39
  diagnosis and [2004], 69
  ethics and, 40
  evaluation and [2004], 74
  identification of issues, problems, and
      trends and, 27
  leadership and, 43
  planning and [2004], 71–72
  quality of practice and, 35
  research and [2004], 81
  resource utilization and, 42
    [2004], 82
  standard of practice for identifying, 27
    [2004], 70
  See also Outcomes identification
Oversight of practice environment, 11,
    16, 17
  as nurse administrator key function, ix,
    2, 10
  organizational, 12

sphere of influence and, 10
  See also Authority of nurse
      administrators

P
Patient
  defined [2004], 84
  ethics and [2004], 79
  evaluation and, 33
  implementation and [2004], 73
  leadership and, 43
  outcome identification [2004], 70
  planning and [2004], 71–72
  quality of care and administrative
      practice [2004], 75
  resource utilization and [2004], 82
Patient care delivery systems [2004], 66
Patient care planning. See Planning
Patient/client/resident (defined) [2004],
    84
Patient Safety: Achieving A New Standard
    of Care (Institute of Medicine), 6–7
Peer review, 37
    [2204], 76
Performance appraisal, standard of
    professional performance [2004],
    55
  See also Professional practice
      evaluation
Personnel. See Human resources
Planning
  identification of issues, problems, and
      trends and, 28
  resource utilization and, 42
  standard of practice, 28
    [2004], 55, 71–72
Practice environments, 9–10
Practice frameworks for nurse
    administrators, 5–9
  appreciative inquiry, 7
  culture of quality and safety, 6–7
  emotional intelligence, 8
  Magnet Recognition Program, 9
  mentoring, 7
  nursing process, 6
  organizational development resources,
    7

transformational leadership (theory
   of), 8
servant leadership (theory of), 8–9
Practice levels. *See* Nurse administrator,
   levels of practice
Preceptors. *See* Mentoring
Privacy. *See* Confidentiality
Problem identification. *See* Diagnosis
Problems and diagnosis, standard of
   practice [2004], 69
   See also Identification of issues,
      problems, and trends
Professional development, 15–17, 19
   collegiality and, 38
   health promotion, health teaching,
      and education, 31
   nurse executive and [2004], 60
   nurse manager and [2004], 64
   professional environment and [2004],
      78
   professional knowledge and [2004], 77
   professional practice evaluation and,
      37
   [2004], 60, 64
   See also Education; Human resources;
      Leadership
Professional environment
   standard of professional performance
      [2004], 55, 78
Professional knowledge, standard of
   professional performance [2004],
      55, *77*
   See also Education; Knowledge base
      of nursing administration
Professional performance. *See*
   Standards of professional
   performance
Professional practice evaluation,
   standard of professional
   performance, 37
   See also Performance appraisal
Program-focused authority (sphere of
   influence), 18
Project-based authority (sphere of
   influence), 18–19
Public and community health, 23
   [2004], 56, 57

Q
Quality of care and administrative practice,
   6–7
   [2004], 55, 75
Quality of practice, 3–14, 17–20 *passim*
   health promotion and, 31
   leadership and, 43
   resource utilization and, 42
   standard of professional performance,
      35
   [2004], 55
   [2004], 58–63 *passim*, 68, 75, 77, 78, 82

R
Recruitment and retention, 5
   nurse executive [2004], 60
   nurse manager and, 16
   [2004], 63, 66
Registered nurse (RN)
   autonomy, 13
   bill of rights, 47
   decision-making and, 15
   recruitment and retention, 16
   See also Nursing
Regulatory and legal compliance, 11, 21,
      24, 28, 33, 35, 37, 40
   [2004], 56, 65, 70, 73, 76, 79
Research, 2
   assessment and [2004], 68
   evaluation and [2004], 78
   nurse executive and [2004], 60–61
   nurse manager and [2004], 64
   planning and [2004], 71
   professional environment and [2004],
      78
   standard of professional
      performance, 41
   [2004], 55, 81
   See also Evidence-based practice
Resident. *See* Patient
Resource utilization
   certification and credentialing [2004],
      82
   education and [2004], 82
   intellectual capital and, 42
   nurse administrator and, 7
   outcome identification and, 42